ENDOI

'Alice knew porn addicte
she wrote *Restored*. In her bc
shares her personal story of porn addiction, trauma, and recovery. Reading *Restored,* you will feel welcomed, seen, known, and cherished. Alice's writing is wise and witty. Her supportive words will make you laugh, cry, and be comforted. You'll know you're not alone. Alice is well informed about the roots of sexual addiction and the steps necessary for healing. She provides many strategies and exercises to propel you forward into a new life. Alice also tackles tough topics that too few Christians talk about. *Restored* will not just help you quit porn. It will give you a hopeful vision for a healthy, shame-free sexuality. You will learn how to develop deep connections with yourself, others, and a loving God. *Restored* is a powerful book. If you're open, it can change your life.'

Forest Benedict, LMFT, SATP, Author of *Life After Lust: Stories & Strategies for Sex & Pornography Addiction Recovery*, ForestBenedict.com.

'This book is a must-read for any woman struggling with porn addiction. Alice has learned a lot on her journey, and the wisdom she shares will provide you with tools that will bring you healing and freedom.'

Brittni De La Mora, Director of XXXChurch.com, author of *Fire: 14 Ways To Keep Your Love On Fire For Him (14 Day Marriage Challenge).*

'Untold numbers of women who struggle in silence and shame will clap, "Me too!" when they read *Restored*. This raw, hopeful, and honest book is a practical recovery guide that also examines the underlying roots for compulsive pornography use and tackles taboo issues like masturbation with nuance and sensitivity.

Restored avoids the rigidity of black-and-white-recovery approaches and goes after a woman's pain-filled heart and her longing for healing. This grace-filled work will resonate with Christian women and with those who struggle to believe in a loving God. I'm so glad to add this terrific resource to my recommendations for female porn and sex addicts!'

Marnie C. Ferree, LMFT, CSAT, Founder and Director of Bethesda Workshops, author of *No Stones: Women Redeemed from Sexual Addiction.*

'When women are excluded from the conversation about porn addiction and recovery, they are shamed into silence. This type of shaming has happened far too often in the mental health and addiction treatment field. Bravo to Alice Taylor for breaking through. Though Alice's take on life and recovery is distinctly Christian, all women who struggle with compulsive porn use will find this book both reassuring and useful.'

Dr. Robert Weiss, Chief Clinical Officer of Seeking Integrity, author of *Sex Addiction 101, Prodependence,* and other books.

Female porn use has been growing exponentially, but with precious few resources specifically targeted at helping women find freedom. Restored is a vulnerable memoir and realistic look at female porn addiction. In her work, Alice Taylor breaks down the walls of shame and restores women to wholeness with insightful advice and wisdom on recovery.

Crystal Renaud Day, MAPC, Founder of Living on Purpose Coaching & Pastoral Counselling and author of *Dirty Girls Come Clean.*

'I once felt *exactly* like Alice about my porn addiction…and about myself. *Restored* beautifully sings into the silence and 'life-draining-shame' that shrouds so many women who struggle with porn. Alice Taylor fills the dark spaces with hope, writing with the authority of one who has been there, suffered, and returned with the resounding gifts of empowered humility and loving service. Thank you Alice for adding this sharply written Christian memoir/workbook to the tiny but growing body of knowledge and inspiration for women with porn problems—I will be referring *Restored* to my clients and colleagues regularly!

Restored is a smart, funny, heart-centered Christian recovery guide for women and everyone who loves them and wants to know what it's like to hurt and heal from porn addiction.'

Staci Sprout, LICSW, CSAT, author of *Naked in Public: A Memoir of Sex Addiction and Other Temporary Insanities.*

'*Restored* is an amazing journey inward, wrought with the wisdom of one whom has travelled the path back to herself, sexually. Alice adds so much to the conversation about women and porn. It's about time we had real advice about these sensitive and timely topics for ourselves, our sisters, and our daughters.'

Lacy Alajna Bentley, Women's recovery coach, author of *Addicted to Love: Recovery, Empowerment and Finding Your True Self.*

'*Restored* offers such a refreshing perspective to the entire porn 'addiction' recovery conversation. Alice's style of writing is forward, blunt, and at times comical but throughout offers deep insight into a topic that has far too long been considered a 'male only' problem. Her advice is practical and comes from personal experience which gives it great weight and merit. Not only does her personal journey offer hope to other women in the same situation, but the advice in this book could apply to anyone who seeks freedom from their pornography use.' **Carl Thomas Jr.**, CEO and founder of Live Free Community App.

Restored

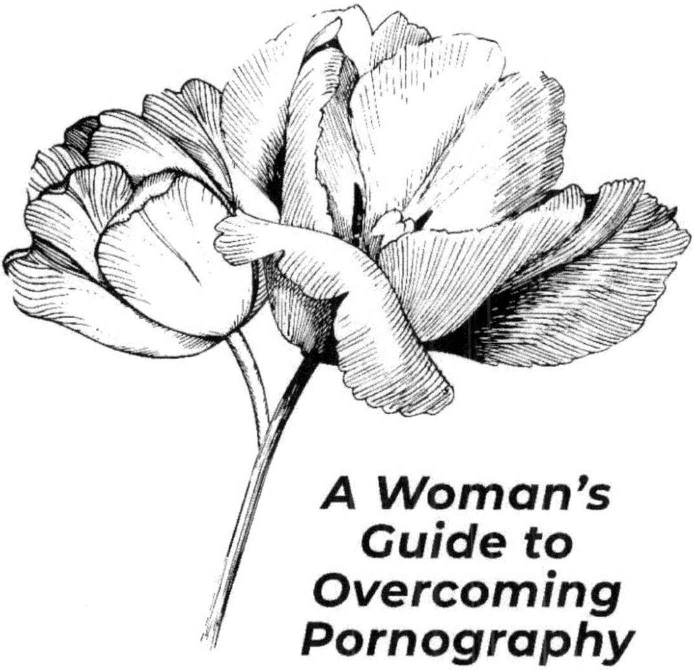

A Woman's Guide to Overcoming Pornography

ALICE TAYLOR

Cover designed by Saffron and Co. Creative.

Thirteen Tulips Publishing. Sydney, Australia.

THIRTEEN
TULIPS
PUBLISHING

All Scripture quotations are taken from the *Holy Bible,* New International Version.

ISBN-13: 978-0-6487220-0-7

Jesus is the author of my story.
What I've done in this book is simply retell what He's done for me and the lessons learnt on the journey. Thank you, Jesus. May you use this book to bring divine healing to many women.

He restores my soul.
Psalm 23:3

TABLE OF CONTENTS

INTRODUCTION

In the depths of my struggle with porn, the Google search bar hosted some truly disturbing requests from yours truly. It was probably just as relieved as I was to have its browser history cleared.

I can just imagine it celebrating when all that sexual content was erased from its memory…until the next time, that is. The thing is, the searches I typed into that little white rectangle that caused the most grief and shame were not the ones which were so desperately seeking intimacy or exploring my wild sexual fantasies but the questions I sent out into the digital abyss.

'How do I stop using porn?'

'How do I stop masturbating?'

'Women + porn addiction'

'Help + women + porn addiction'

'Do women watch porn?'

'Porn addiction recovery + women'

'Christian women who struggle with porn'

'Porn help for women'

… 'What's wrong with me?'

These questions, along with my favourite porn websites, haunted my browser history. Are they familiar to you too? Chances are, you've searched for the same things and probably came across the same frustrating, confusing and disappointing results—everything is for men. If an article, book or recovery website happened to mention women, it was usually for wives of porn addicts. It was a rarity to find a website or resource specifically created for women struggling with porn.

When women are excluded from the conversation on recovery, they are shamed into silence. They feel alone. This is where the real, life-draining shame thrives. You and I both know this. And it's not only the internet that is lacking. Almost every time the topic of porn is tentatively broached in Church, it's for 'the guys' while women are given talks on modesty and relationships. Most books about pornography are drowning in masculine pronouns, blogs are directed at male addicts and feminist organisations emphasise the male-oriented nature of porn. Everything is for 'him' and this makes 'her' feel like a freak.

The current narrative of porn being a male issue drains women who struggle of their sense of femininity and worth. When I was struggling the most, I felt undesirable, worthless, unlovable and, frankly, disgusting. I felt so much shame from my porn use, and it was made worse by the total and utter silence surrounding the topic. I truly believed I was alone. I felt I was better off hiding, keeping this secret locked away. I thought the pain and shame I was already living with was enough without any more being added.

This book is for every woman who has ever felt this way. I wrote this guide in response to the echoing silence surrounding the topic of women and porn, to break the stigma that only men struggle with it, and to open up a healing conversation about the unique needs of women recovering from pornography addiction. *Restored* is your practical recovery guide, based off my own story of addiction and finding freedom.

What you will read in the coming ten chapters are the step-by-step basics to beginning your journey in overcoming porn. To get the most out of this book, I recommend doing an initial read-through before implementing any of the Action Steps. This can be a simple skim read but enough to give yourself an idea of where you're headed.

Once your head is in the game and you're ready to go, read each chapter at a steady pace and practice the recommended activities as they come. I suggest finding yourself a nice new journal full of blank pages to write your reflections in, and to expand on the Action Steps which follow each chapter. If you start to feel overwhelmed by the ever-growing recovery 'to-do' list, take a break and focus on the current step until it's more familiar, before moving on to the next chapter.

I'm so excited for you to journey through *Restored*! Not only will this guide provide you with advice on how to find freedom, but it will encourage you to pursue restoration. It is my hope you will find yourself and your true tribe. Recovery isn't simply about learning how to restrict negative behaviours, it is equally about reconnecting with yourself, your community, God and the world. It's about creating a life you love, a life you don't want to escape from anymore. Recovery is like a train track, you have two parallel rails pointing in the same direction, one is sobriety and the other is restoration. Together they move you forward.

Unfortunately, this is not achievable overnight. You won't experience restoration by simply picking up this book and hoping it will fix you, either. To overcome the shackles of habitual porn use or masturbation and flourish in your everyday life is no simple task. This will take time and commitment. Recovery takes more than just desire for healing, but the strength to put what you learn into action, to follow through with conviction and do the things that scare the pants off you.

I want to be honest with you right from the get-go: this journey will not be easy. It will push you to your limits and ask you to do things you never imagined you would, but the reward is great. By pushing through fear and doing something new with your life, you will learn so much! You will grow in character, you will meet new people who will become friends for life, and you will experience freedom like you never thought possible in your darkest days. What you've been doing thus far hasn't worked too well, has it? That's why you're here, reading this, instead of living out your freedom. So, give this process a chance, even when it gets tough. It won't be easy, but it will be worth it. You've got nothing to lose, except a porn problem.

With that said, be strong, but be gentle on yourself. Take this journey at your own pace. There are no bonus points for reading this book the fastest! This book is intended to be held onto, to be revisited and poured over with care. People say the Bible has a new message for them no matter how many times they read the same story—I'm not saying *Restored* has been possessed by the Holy Spirit, but I do hope with each new season you enter during recovery you can come back to this guide and find something new to reflect and work on. I hope as you grow deeper in self-awareness and healing you can take your recovery to new heights. Rest your heart and mind as you need, pick up a journal and write or draw out your thoughts, have a big, fat cry, talk it out with a friend or mentor, and never forget the healing power of naps!

This book is also not to be read with perfection in mind, but rather with a good dose of realism. You won't get everything right; in fact, I don't want you to! Making mistakes is part of healing, it's something you should expect. This is not permission to throw caution to the wind and give up before you start but be prepared to treat yourself with kindness and forgiveness and move on if (when) you do mess-up. In imperfection, we are given an opportunity to step back, reflect and change. A slip-up in any part of life is only a failure if you don't learn from it. Pursue success but embrace mistakes on the journey.

I wonder how you feel after reading this introduction. As I write this, sun shining through my balcony window, covering my pyjama-clad legs in a warm glow, I feel vulnerable. This whole book is the biggest risk I've ever taken. I'm baring my deepest soul to the whole world and inviting strangers into my private story. I think my words might make you feel this way, too. Do you feel vulnerable holding this book with the words 'pornography' and 'woman' slapped on the front in bold purple font? This might be the first time you've pulled off that good-Christian-girl mask and admitted you have a problem with porn. How does it feel to be honest and admit your darkness? It's probably a bit overwhelming, and a lot scary. I remember what it feels like, and I know you've taken a huge step in being here for yourself, now. I'm proud of you. Picking up this book takes courage.

I didn't have a step-by-step guide like this when I was struggling. I wish I had. My recovery was a haphazard journey through highs, lows and painful frustration which spanned over ten years. I have been imperfect in my healing—I've lied, manipulated like only an addict knows how, experienced temporary lapses and major relapses. My story has a happy ending though. I live a fulfilled life full of healthy relationships, I know real joy and freedom, and am no longer a slave to the screen. I am happily married and enjoy mutually fulfilling sexual intimacy with my husband. I live with so much less fear these days, and when troubled times come, I have the resources to deal with my issues in healthy ways. To be honest, I can still be a train-wreck! I'm not perfect. But the difference now is I have a safe community supporting me, I trust Jesus and know the bad times will pass by the time we arrive at the next station. My life is radically different today compared to when I first started this recovery journey, I can barely believe it. But don't take my word for it, read on and see for yourself.

The names and details of people mentioned throughout this book may have been altered for their privacy, and are all used with permission.

CHAPTER ONE: MY STORY

There are a lot of dark places pornography can take a woman. However, I never anticipated one of the lowest moments during my addiction to porn would involve setting an oven on fire trying to cook pasta.

Porn ruins everything; *of course* it would try to ruin my delicious bowl of cheesy carbs.

Let me explain.

In my late teens and early twenties, I was a prime candidate for house and pet sitting. Elderly couples and families from church would offer me residence in their homes for weeks at a time while they holidayed. I had the chance to get away from my family, experience freedom and give the holiday makers some peace of mind and security. I was the obvious choice for them, I was kind and softly spoken, I worked in children's ministry and attended Bible college. I was young, single and absolutely lovely. Little did they know it wasn't the out-of-home experience I cherished, the independence from my parents or even the cash that sometimes came with the job, but rather the freedom it granted me to indulge in pornography and frequent masturbation without the risk of being caught.

One particular couple had me stay at their large house while they were away in Japan. I spent the entire weekend indulging in pornography and masturbating as much as I pleased, only to come crashing down in a porn hangover by Monday. You probably know exactly what I'm talking about, but for those yet to experience the unique crap-storm that is a porn hangover, it's a dreadful combination of regret, shame, anger and helplessness that manifests in physical, emotional, mental and spiritual ways. It feels very similar to an alcohol comedown, but instead of splattered vomit, you spend the morning cleaning up your browser history.

That's where I found myself on that Monday morning, shame gripping my entire body. I felt disgusted at what I had done, which was only amplified by the homely environment I found myself in. Who watches hardcore porn while surrounded by doyleys and creepy china dolls? (I do). What would these people think if they knew how I had used my time? I anticipated their judgement and let it sink deep into my skin as punishment. I deserved to be rejected and damned.

I found myself lying in the foetal position in the middle of their greenhouse. Amongst delicate ferns and moss, I fell apart.

'I. Can't. Stop! What have I become?'

The edges of my soul felt as if they were shrinking up within me. Like a worn-out jumper, threads were coming loose, pulling me up into nothing.

After a few numb hours staring at a particularly ugly plant and contemplating how my life was falling apart, the only solution I could think of was to get up, brush the dust off myself, raid the alcohol stash, drink too much, and cook myself some pity-pasta. It turns out I forgot to remove the metal cover off the heated element before slamming my pot of pasta on top of it. After a few hours of confusion and abuse from me, the whole thing exploded in flames.

My week didn't get much better after that.

Somehow, I managed to buy replacement parts for the old-fashioned oven on eBay and hide the charred evidence before the couple got home. Nevertheless, it was still a low-light. You could call it my rock-bottom (or one of many if we're being honest).

Unfortunately, I didn't rally from this soon after. I fell into a deep, hateful depression, and let my mind wander into other worlds. There were many a night where I seriously considered where I could find drugs or sex to salve this pain I was feeling and escape reality. I count myself very blessed to have missed the Tinder boat by a few years, and to have had some intervention before any of these wandering thoughts became a reality.

So how does a quiet little Christian girl with a bowl-cut grow up to be an oven-destroying porn addict?

It all began when I was just twelve years old. Our family was lacking in the sex education department. I have two memories of learning about sex, the first was a 'How are babies made?' cartoon my brother and I watched on our old VHS player, and the second was an innocent question little Alice chirped up with from the back seat of our family car, as we were driving Grandma home.

'Mum, what does horny mean?' I asked. I can only imagine the panic on my poor mother's face as she drove along the highway. To her credit, she calmly responded that it meant someone was ready to have sex.

She then asked, 'Where did you hear that?'. She must have been relieved when I calmly explained that it was a new insult going around the school yard. I'm proud of my mum for being so calm and real in these instances, and providing my brother and I with a basic education—even if she did outsource it to a cartoon couple with soap suds hanging off their private parts who, for some reason, deemed it necessary to explain that babies didn't arrive in burgers or oversized hats.

As my brother and I got older, the conversations seemed to stop. Or at least they became more rigid and question avoidant. Rules were put in place in our household without appropriate explanation of why. For example, the old open-door policy when boyfriends or girlfriends visited. In hindsight, I think it's a great rule, and one which I'll be employing when I have my own children. But I intend to calmly sit down with my kids and explain why it's a rule, share my own experience and allow them to push back and ask questions. It'll be a discussion, not a brick wall boxing them in.

The Bible was my parents' guide and it felt like any questions about their interpretation were an offence against God Himself. The mantra in our household was 'Because the Bible says so!'. This was a stock-standard answer to many healthy curiosities about sexuality and other 'controversial' topics which only served to shut down genuine discussion and made me feel unheard and frustrated. I wanted to understand the world; instead I had a Bible lobbed at my face. Their 'biblical' responses seemed one-dimensional and out of touch with reality. They only left me feeling more confused and ill-at-ease with Christianity.

So, at twelve years old, when I stumbled upon soft-core porn (on good old dial-up internet) it started to fill the blanks. It satisfied my curiosities better than my parents did, and I was totally fascinated by this new online world of naked bodies. I explored some of the new sexual things I was learning with a random guy from America, who I met online. Our digital characters would make out, and we'd have childish but sexually suggestive chats. When I was offline, I scoured novels for steamy sex scenes and even took these books on family holidays to read over and over again.

I had no idea what I was watching was pornography, or what I was doing was called masturbation and cybersex. In fact, I'd never even heard those words before! Sex between a married couple was barely on the table for conversation in our home, so the porn and online safety talk had no chance. In the nineties I don't think my parents knew themselves the threat cyberspace posed to young boys and girls.

This was the first stepping stone into addiction. With the discovery of pornography, and the puberty hormones pumping through my system, I was in a constant state of arousal. Sex was on my mind 24/7 and I took every chance I had to be alone with a computer, erotic novel or my own thoughts. A few birthdays down the track though, I ceased my online searching and chatting for a few years. The high school experience was about to take over my life and change me in more ways than I could ever imagine. The next phase of my life story has less to do with sex, and everything to do with the pain that set me up for an adult life of porn addiction and dysfunctional behaviour.

I was bullied. It was intense, relentless and cruel. For two years of my life, I lived in fear. At my notoriously rough school, my small group of friends and I were singled out as the 'weirdos' and 'misfits'. Name calling, taunting, getting spat on and rumour spreading were the norm. It didn't stop at the school gates either. The sound of a person screaming insults out of a moving car is familiar, and unexpected yelling in the streets still puts me on high alert. My best friend, the eccentric emo boy I dated and I all experienced physical abuse, too. Besides being spat on, we have been in headlocks, threatened with physical violence and had cigarettes and glass bottles thrown at us in public. The worst experience by far was when my boyfriend was horribly assaulted by two guys waiting for us at his house. I was devastated and terrified—this was the bloody cherry on top of a horrible, traumatic sundae. I was later diagnosed with Post Traumatic Stress Disorder from these events, but that diagnosis and subsequent treatment didn't happen until I was in my twenties.

I powered through undiagnosed and untreated mental illness for another five years. It was tough. I didn't know what was wrong with me, but knew something wasn't right. I was unstable, emotional and vulnerable.

School wasn't my only source of pain. There was tension in my household which kept me locked in an anxious, depressed and often vengeful mindset.

I felt disconnected from my family, which only increased as my mental health deteriorated and I spiralled into another dimension of pain and secrecy. I resented them for my sheltered and odd upbringing, and blamed them for the direction my life was taking, which was messy, scary and lonely. With the relentless bullying at school and feeling constantly unsafe, I couldn't deal with the tension at home as well. My dad was unwell and living with a spinal injury, and Mum had to pick up the slack as well as being a busy primary school teacher and parent to two angry teenagers. Arguments happened, stress boiled over. I hated it.

There was a lot of rage during this time. A lot of screaming and yelling, from both my parents and me. Once, I even punched a hole in my dad's bedroom door. I buried knives deep into my bedroom walls and dragged them through the plaster wishing it was flesh (mine or someone else's ... I couldn't tell). My only refuge in this stormy home was my older brother, who seemed to understand the chaos in my heart. He understood the feelings of resentment and rebellion. He noticed my pain and he cared. He did not abandon me in my time of need, as I felt everyone else had.

Eventually, my parents moved me to a different school for my Higher School Certificate and realised I needed professional counselling to deal with my raging emotions. These two things changed my life, and are the reason I'm a fairly functional, happy woman today. I am so, so grateful for these interventions, even though as a teenager I resented them. Despite all these positive changes though, I was still wounded. I was still vulnerable, and desperate for affection and intimacy.

I searched for these things in all the wrong places. I thought they were only available through a man's approval. After graduating year twelve, I entered into a long-distance relationship with a near-stranger from New Zealand, who didn't share my developing Christian beliefs. My family didn't approve, which I kind of liked.

After several visits back and forth, we decided to become exclusive. And not long after that, despite knowing I wanted to wait until marriage, he pressured me into having sex. He wore me down and convinced me I had very little value besides my ability to please him. Even in that aspect he made me well aware I was incompetent. My body was not up to standard, and I was humiliated into changing myself to satisfy him.

There was no intimacy in what we did. There was never a moment where I felt cared for, nurtured or valued. I barely even felt desired. There was a distinct lack of eye-contact, there was much more aggression than necessary and he did not once consider my pleasure as important. He told me I was 'forgettable' and pushed me aside once he was done with me. A friend watched this relationship play out from a distance. Finally, he could no longer bear the damage being done to my heart, and suggested I break up with Mr Long-Distance. I was so unempowered in myself, I didn't think this was even an option. My Kiwi 'lover' made sure to instil a sense of incompetency and dependence in me. I was chained to him for worth. But my insightful and kind friend who lived in the same country as me spoke the words that gave me courage to break free. He told me I deserved to be loved and cared for, not mistreated.

Unbeknownst to us, our God had a much larger plan in play. Seven long years later, this truly platonic friendship developed into a relationship. Not long after this, Lukas would propose to me on a beautiful mountain top and finally call me his wife. Isn't God's timing and provision so wonderful and generous?

Before that joy would come along however, I had many years of struggle and healing ahead.

With the momentary courage gifted to me by Lukas (and with some coaching over online chat), I ended things with the boy. This was good. With the wisdom of hindsight, I no longer believe he had harmful intentions. This eighteen-year-old boy had a very misguided and damaged understanding of sex and relationships. I can now see this as the result of his pornography use, which he was very open about, and his particular friendship group who certainly didn't champion morality or respect for women. Nevertheless, that relationship became the force that threw me back into the arms of pornography, in a more damaging way than ever before. Once single again, I had space to feel my repressed emotions, and ask the unnerving questions:

Why was sex so terrible?

What was wrong with me?

What did I do wrong?!

… And what was an orgasm, for that matter?

I quickly rediscovered masturbation and pornography in my seeking…But this was not the soft-core pornography of my younger years. The whole landscape of porn had changed radically by the time I was returning to it at eighteen. It was more accessible, acceptable and intense than I had ever seen before. Not to mention, I now owned my own smart phone, laptop and had high speed internet. If I got hooked before, I had no chance this time around.

It began as an education. Like my twelve-year-old self, I still felt sexually naïve despite my new sexual experience. I wanted to understand what sex was supposed to look like, to figure out what I was missing. I used porn as a way of learning what a woman was supposed to look like, act like and do during sex. What did men want? I was preparing for 'next time'. I couldn't bear to be humiliated again at my most vulnerable.

It started off with risqué articles or blogs, I sought advice and frequented blogs that would take reader questions on sexuality and answer them. Sometimes these would have X-rated pictures or GIFs in them, and these grabbed my attention. I began to focus on websites that had more of these images or short videos. They drew me in. My curiosity was insatiable, and there was no question I was aroused. Soon, they weren't enough to give me that familiar rush though, and I tentatively dipped my toe into the big wide world of video pornography.

Here, I found a whole new syllabus for what I was trying to learn! My vocabulary grew, as did my dependence on these explicit videos. I discovered a never-ending source of sex education, and I liked it.

It wasn't long before all thoughts of education and learning faded away. Instead, porn became my escape. It was a fantasy world I could slip away into whenever I pleased. If I didn't have access to a screen, I had a growing memory bank of images in my mind, which were far too easy to conjure at a moment's notice.

I fantasised I was the woman in the video. I was sexy, desired and wanted. All I craved was affection and affirmation, and I falsely sought this by imagining I was desirable for sex. In my mind, I swapped out the nameless actors and actresses for my ex-boyfriend and me. In this fantasy world we were having good, enjoyable sex. He wanted me, I sent him crazy, and I was never, ever told how terrible or ugly I was. There was no risk of rejection in this world and I felt like I got all the benefits of 'intimacy' without the junk.

Sex was the only language I knew. All that romance and love business was just something made up by desperate girls and stupid chick flicks, right? At this point, sex was lord and true romantic love and intimacy were a myth to me. I struggled to believe it was real. There is no such thing as love, only sex.

First it was an education, then it was an escape. Next, it became an addiction.

I discovered porn was a great anaesthetic for pain.

Not only the pain of ruptured intimacy and shame from the ex-boyfriend, but it effectively medicated my wounds from my sheltered and confused upbringing, the bullying and abuse I suffered during high school and the ever-increasing tension in my family home. Not to mention the growing shame I felt about using porn so compulsively.

At the time, I felt like it effectively combated the intense shame and self-hatred I felt towards myself. The rush of dopamine made me feel alive for a few moments, and it made me feel 'in control' when I felt lost and vulnerable. However, the inevitable porn hangover would arrive after a session and I would feel everything I felt previously ... but with an even higher dose of shame and pain. I ended up trapped in a deadly and addictive cycle. I certainly was not in control.

My life became consumed with a combination of increasingly graphic porn, and a shame that covered every fibre of my being. I tried to stop. I couldn't. I had become chemically and emotionally dependent. The shame grew heavier. I felt I couldn't tell anybody. Because porn is a guy's issue, right?

Once I finally realised I had a problem, I did what every millennial would do. I googled it. Hundreds of articles, videos, sermons, books and recovery resources appeared. Some of my searches accidentally led me to more porn, but even more harmful was the complete dominance of male pronouns.

If the *internet* wasn't talking about women and porn addiction, it must be bad, I thought. Really, really bad. I must be a freak. I truly thought I was the only woman watching it and struggling to stop. It remained my secret for many years. That was, until I was graciously given another opportunity to break free. During a Sunday church service the pastor spoke on recurring sin and shame. Without mentioning pornography at all, the Holy Spirit used his words to minister to my soul. I felt an overwhelming sense of love and being known. That evening, I knew God saw deep into my soul and mind. He saw every struggle and image, and still loved me.

I fell to the floor in tears. God was showing me it was time to surrender my addiction to him, and I was so ready. I was terrified, but exhausted from the duplicity of it all. I couldn't do anything but sob uncontrollably.

In a church amphitheatre holding a few hundred people, one woman came to me. I had never met or even seen her before. She held me and prayed healing into my soul. Through guttural sobs, I revealed my secret for the first time. It was terrifying and liberating. I knew God had sent her to me when she responded by confessing she, too, had once struggled with promiscuity, pornography addiction and the unique shame of being a woman hooked. This was my first taste of hope in many years. She had overcome!

This God-sent woman encouraged and empowered me to share my struggle with my best friend, too. She said I needed on the ground accountability, and I needed to fight against secrecy. I needed to be vulnerable in order to heal. I was so scared to take her advice. It took me hours to summon the courage but eventually I confided in my closest friend. Again, I was blown away by the kindness of God as she responded in shocked joy. 'Me too!' she said, to my surprise. 'I thought I was the only one!'

So, the long and arduous road to recovery began. And I had a mentor and friend to walk with me, encourage me, and kick my butt. But I'll be honest: Getting free from porn hurt like hell. It took years of relapses and painful confessions to truly find freedom. It took counselling, prayer, accountability, filtering software, tears and hard work. I had to deal with my PTSD and every wound that fed the intimacy disorder I had developed. It hurt.

Throughout the mess, Jesus loved me. He never stopped showing me kindness, even at my darkest. His Holy Spirit showed me gentle and persistent love in unique and undeniable ways. He told me that He knew it all and still cherished me! He taught me that my struggle didn't diminish my femininity or worth. As I received this love, my shame began to seep away. My intimacy with both God and those around me was restored. This healing paved the way for me to use the tools I had to truly seek freedom.

It wasn't easy. Having God on your side doesn't instantly solve every problem. But it does mean you know grace. It means you know acceptance and unconditional love, even in your darkest hour.

Today, I am married to an incredible man who knows my entire journey. We enjoy a thriving sex life, and I rest assured knowing I am completely known and loved, not only by him, but by God too. There have been several times in the last few years when I've lapsed and used pornography, even while writing this book and happily married. The difference between then and now though, is that these occurrences are only a few times a year, not daily. I'm now able to bounce back from a lapse and reflect on what triggered it, and confidently share my mistake with Lukas, my accountability partner, and sometimes the whole internet through my website The Grace Spot and move forward. I may experience lapses sometimes, but I no longer live in shame. My relationship with God, my parents, those around me and my own body have drastically improved, and I live in the joy of that freedom, and grow more whole and shameless every passing day.

CHAPTER TWO: ACCOUNTABILITY

An invitation to be courageous

I'm going to ask you to do something brave. I'm going to ask you to look your addiction right in the face, and do the opposite of what it tells you to do. You're going to tell someone what's going on.

You're freely going to confess you are a woman enslaved to pornography and in pain. Not only am I asking you to tell someone how you're *really* going, but you're going to keep telling someone how you're going. This is accountability, and it is the first step to your restoration.

Now, I know this is the exact thing you've been working your whole life to avoid. Telling someone your secret feels like unravelling a tightly and meticulously knitted ball you have fought so hard to keep hidden! That's exactly what it is, though. I'm inviting you to unravel ... but not on your own.

You're going to start pulling at those threads and working through them until they come loose. And the very first thing you're going to need to pull at is your life of secrecy. If you want to heal, you've got to undo this by confessing your struggle and getting accountable.

Why you need this

If you're anything like me, you'll have read the previous paragraph while turning the cogs in your brain to figure out some creative way to do the whole recovery thing *without* this accountability. In the beginning, all I wanted was a way out and, like a toddler unhappy about having to eat her greens, I cried, 'BUT WHY?! Do I have to?'

Asking 'why' is a good thing though, because there are some convincing reasons why you really and truly *do* need accountability. It's also a good opportunity for you to be honest with yourself. I mean, really—if you *could* overcome pornography addiction on your own, you wouldn't be here, would you? You'd have dealt with it on your own, and be skipping through a field of daisies by now. If you're asking why and would rather avoid this step, I get it. But your ongoing struggle should be all the evidence you need to realise it's a necessity.

I know it sucks but this is your welcome to the realm of recovery, where the right thing to do is the thing you no-way-in-hell want to do, and where healing comes from excavating and enduring pain. It's unfortunate, it's not easy; but let me fill you in on a little recovery secret…

When you feel resistance, when you want to pull away and hide, that means you're making progress. If you're coming up against a step that makes you uncomfortable, and you want to run in the opposite direction—that's a signal to push forward.

Why?

Addiction wants to survive. It will do its best to pull you back into the darkness. It will whisper lies and stir up painful emotions in an attempt to silence your courageous assault against it. It will exploit your fears and turn them into panic, all in order to keep you in its hold. The voice that tells you to back down from honesty and integrity isn't yours, it's addiction begging you not to eradicate it. It has made quite a comfortable home within you, and it wants to stay! But you're the landlord, and you get to kick out tenants who damage your precious property (that's you!).

If kicking addiction right in the face doesn't give you enough reason to fully commit to the accountability process, there are some other vital reasons you need it, too.

The brain on autopilot

We'll discuss the impact of pornography on the brain more in chapter five, but simply put, when you're addicted to pornography, your brain is on autopilot. At this point, it's moved from a simple 'moral failing' or 'bad habit', to something that is out of your control. Even if you don't know much about the science behind porn addiction, I'm sure you've experienced this out-of-control feeling. You see, porn activates the reward pathway in your brain to release a host of feel-good-sexual-high chemicals that under medical observation, appear remarkably similar to the chemicals involved when a user takes drugs. Your brain thrives off these and doesn't want to let go. One taste, and it's hooked. It's taking you all the way through your acting out process. This isn't to say you have zero control over your actions, but it's tough as hell to resist that biological urge. This is why you need someone on the outside. You need another brain on your team! One that isn't flooded with sex chemicals and desire in the moment of your temptation. You need someone to lovingly speak logic and reason into your life when you and your brain are overcome.

An accountability partner can be a friend or an older, wiser mentor in your life. Whoever you choose, consider them like a personal trainer for your brain. Anyone who's ever tried to lose weight or tone up will attest to the difficulty of staying motivated and on track on their own.

Many of us have a stash of gym key codes or free sweat towels stashed at the bottom of some forgotten drawer in our house. It's just not easy. Our body and mind don't want to eat broccoli and run on a treadmill for hours. It's not the lifestyle we're used to, and our brains haven't yet made the connection that healthy living is more rewarding than neglecting ourselves.

Have you ever forked out the extra cash for a PT? I have. It took sacrifice, in terms of finances and actual commitment to training, but boy, oh boy did it pay off! Before I had a trainer to keep me accountable, I would fall off the wagon within weeks or months. But with a trainer who was stronger, fitter and more committed to pushing me than I was, I made the most progress I've ever made. I told him my values and goals at the start of our partnership. I wanted to lose weight, get stronger and eat better. He held me accountable to these by asking me each and every week how I was doing, by writing me programs specific to my goals and calling me out when I slacked off. It was powerful. When my brain said 'No, I don't wanna work hard today!', he said, 'Just do it anyway. I'm watching!'.

With someone on the outside supporting me, I succeeded. Instead of finding myself elbow deep in a bucket of Kentucky Fried Chicken after a few weeks of haphazard treadmilling and starving myself, I achieved my goals. My newfound success felt like a miracle, but in reality, it was just accountability doing its job.

The 'why' of accountability goes beyond the need to have an outside source kick your brain back into reality and help you achieve your goals, however. There's more. Accountability is about restoring intimacy and healing, too.

Addiction is isolating. The unique blend of shame, despair and preoccupation with a behaviour or substance turns people inward and puts them into hiding. If they're not physically absent and lacking community, women are often emotionally vacant in their friendships and limited in their ability to be vulnerable, honest and real.

As you participate in accountability, you'll get a side order of healing. Accountability relationships play an important role in developing your ability to relate to others and share genuine connection without shame or sex. They may be the first safe place you've ever known, and this lays the foundation for relearning healthy intimacy.

As difficult as it may feel going from zero-to-sixty in the vulnerability department with a female friend, it is such a vital thing to relearn for a sustained recovery. Healthy, whole and honest female friendships will be vital to restoring you to the woman you truly are underneath your struggle. It's been said that the opposite of addiction is connection, and it begins with this single, vital relationship.

Dispelling the myths

Now you have the information on why you need accountability, but does it still make you feel queasy? Is all this giving you butterflies in your stomach? It's okay if accountability scares you; it's not a familiar practice and new things can be intimidating.

I think part of that fear also comes from distorted views of what accountability actually is … and what it isn't. Accountability isn't about shame. This process isn't about sitting across from someone as a guilty party or judge, and it's definitely not about shaming someone out of their behaviours. Accountability isn't compiling a big list of sins and paying for them. It's not an opportunity to be harsh on yourself or have someone else be harsh on you. In our individualistic society so focused on personal happiness, and with tolerance held in such high esteem, it seems accountability is a lost art. Having a friend pull you up on inconsistencies or mistakes is seen as judgemental and associated with negativity. Admitting you want to change your behaviours and asking for help to be more consistent in your beliefs and actions can be perceived as being brain-washed (by a religion, tradition or family, etc.). Our culture doesn't like it. The prevailing belief is that you should be 'true to yourself', i.e. do what your 'heart' or emotions tell you. In general, it seems accountability has a 'Big Brother' vibe in our society, and is not something understood, celebrated or practiced.

This is such a shame, because real accountability is uplifting. Instead of being an opportunity to judge and condemn, it's an opening for grace and healing. It's a safe place to be unapologetically you and receive affirmation and love. It's a way of delving deep and investing in a friendship that speaks truth and love. Not only this, but it's an effective and joyful way to become a better version of you! Accountability isn't all about the doom and gloom of failed goals, but is also about celebrating your victories and successes with a trusted friend or mentor. It's not a reaction to getting caught out, but it's proactive living, putting everything out in the open and being free in that.

Can you imagine a life truly free from secrets, with at least one other person? Can you imagine not having the anxiety and fear that comes with holding in secrets and hiding part of yourself? Can you picture yourself experiencing that kind of freedom with someone? That depth of intimacy? How great does that sound?!

Accountability isn't a cage intended to trap and torture you—it's a safety net that allows you to soar higher than you ever thought possible.

Now I'm done drumming the necessity of accountability into your head, it's time to move on to the practical. The following information will be your accountability roadmap. We'll be focusing on who to share your struggle with and the six pillars of successful and lasting accountability.

Who to tell?

Let's start with that all-important question: Who are you going to tell? How do you turn a regular relationship into an accountability one without flopping into a pile of goop on the floor and freaking out?

First, you need a woman you can trust with your heart. Yes, women only! Trying to do accountability with a guy will only confuse boundaries and get messy; stick with your own kind. I'd recommend the same for same-sex attracted women, because although you may not feel any kind of romantic intimacy or temptation sharing your sexual struggles with a man, he might. That said, same-sex attracted women should avoid striking up an accountability partnership with a woman they are romantically interested in. This too can become messy due to the intimate nature of your conversations. Amy Riordan, author of *Longing for Intimacy*[1] and vocal advocate for women struggling with both pornography and same-sex attraction recommends seeking out an older female mentor to be accountable with. If sharing your temptations with her or anyone else is becoming a trigger, take a step back and seek support elsewhere.

Straight or LGBTQI+, you need to identify a woman who has shown herself to be trustworthy, safe and kind.

The woman you want to share your heart with should have a solid history of being non-judgemental, loving, accepting and compassionate. This responsibility isn't for the faint of heart, either. Your chosen confidant should be someone with mental determination and grit, along with grace. When considering someone to tell, ask yourself, is she someone who would keep me honest? Would she stand up to my excuses and questionable behaviour? Does she have just enough sass or tough-mum-love to keep me on track when I try to wander away?

It's great to have a few women you can talk to about these issues. You may have one primary accountability partner, but it doesn't hurt to have a few girlfriends on speed dial when you can't get in touch with your main gal or she's dealing with her own mess. No one is going to be available 24/7. Does anyone come to mind?

If you have a husband or partner, they cannot stand in this place. Yes, you need to disclose your addiction to them. Yes, you need to remain in open conversation about both of your emotions and needs. But telling an intimate partner of every temptation and lapse would send them insane. It would break their heart over and over and make for a fairly unhealthy relationship. You need to tell your partner, but you also need at least one woman on the outside to support you.

What if I don't have any close female friends?

It can be tough juggling a porn addiction and any kind of relationship, let alone complex female friendships. You may not have anyone who comes to mind when I say 'trusted woman or friend'.

If you struggle to think of someone, consider any female connections you do have. Is there someone safe from your church community you can contact? Could you speak to a pastoral care worker or minister about connecting with a caring woman in your community? You would be surprised just how many older women are desperate to mentor younger ones. Perhaps there is a woman in your life you are no longer close with, but you know her character is loving and safe. Could you take the courage to reconnect and ask her for help? You never know where it may lead. Alternatively, are there any support groups in your area that cater to women with sexual addictions? Can you access an online support group? These are places which work whole programs together, but also provide community and accountability.

If you still find yourself scratching your head after all this pondering, there are a number of female sexual addiction recovery coaches available online as well as professional counsellors who may be able to support you. It's best to engage with someone who is part of your daily life (bonus: it's free!) but if you must, there is temporary accountability available to get you started. You can find more information about recovery coaches and where to access them on The Grace Spot.

Figuring out who to confess to is one thing, but then you need to actually do it. To find encouragement, advice and inspiration, you can head to The Grace Spot to browse blogs and personal accounts from women who have bravely gone before you in confession. The two most important things to remember though, are these: There's no exact format or script you must follow. Adjust the conversation to suit your story, communication style and relationship with whoever you're sharing with. And second, know that you might not ever overcome the fear of confession before you do it. Don't wait until you feel confident, because you may never speak. Sharing your struggle is scary. It's requires huge vulnerability, which is probably an unfamiliar behaviour. You don't need to eradicate fear in order to have this conversation, you just need to be brave.

What does accountability look like on the ground?

By far the most common question I'm asked once that initial confession is out of the way and the other party agrees to walk this journey with you is 'what should accountability actually look like?'. Accountability is a unique relationship and will look different for everyone. Some women like to sit down in a quiet place with coffee, while others may do accountability best on horseback or through Skype at midnight. There is no exact formula, however there are six pillars of accountability that should form the foundation of any relationship. We'll be examining each of these in detail but there's something you must do before getting into the details.

An alcoholic won't recover sitting in a bar, the drug addict who keeps a stash in her room is doomed and someone trying to quit smoking is only causing themselves pain by spending all their time in a cloud of others' smoke. You know this. The same goes for the porn addict—if you want to find freedom you must purge yourself of porn, and anything that causes you to stumble.

This includes erotic novels, magazines, any hidden folders containing porn on your computer, subscriptions to websites and anything else that brings porn into your life. If you use a vibrator or other sex toy when you watch porn, it's time to say goodbye to them, too. You *know* that's only going to be a temptation. This process also includes a social media detox. These are refreshing at the best of times, but this one is going to be particularly helpful for your healing. Unfollow, block or delete any person or pages that tempt you. These may be accounts that share sexual content, images that make you feel less-than and ashamed about your body (I'm looking at you, fitspo!), anything that makes you feel down about yourself and anything that makes you feel drained, anxious, frustrated or depressed. If you're going to spend time online, make sure you fill your feeds with positivity and light. If social media still feels a little out of control for you after doing a detox, maybe it's time to take a break for a while. I'm totally on board with this; taking a break from endlessly scrolling through cyberspace will only benefit your wellbeing!

Next up, it's time for software. If you are a woman struggling with online pornography, you need filtering software. There are free and paid options which work on iPhones, androids, PCs and laptops, so you have no excuse not to have it. These have the ability to block specific and general pornographic websites, and many have a reporting feature which sends an email to a trusted friend listing all the websites visited on your computer in the last week or two. Scary stuff, huh? But you know you need it. Find my personal recommendations for filtering software on The Grace Spot, listed under 'Get Help' followed by 'Restrict Access'.

The six pillars of great accountability

1. *Responsibility*

Both accountability partners have responsibilities. But first and foremost, you must take responsibility for yourself. Accountability isn't going to do you any favours if you're not honest. And that starts with you.

You must be prepared to break through any excuses, ...tion or plain lies that want to come out. Trust me, they will. This doesn't make you a bad or manipulative person, it just means you're a recovering person. As you grow more and more into recovery, you will get better at identifying unhelpful thoughts and internal justifications. At first, it can be difficult. It never ceases to amaze me just how legitimate our internal excuses can be. You can even fool yourself.

You run the risk of sabotaging your recovery by shifting responsibility onto others, especially when it comes to accountability. When I asked a small group of recovering women their greatest struggle with accountability, most of them said they wished their friends who knew would check in on them more frequently. This is not taking personal responsibility. Taking responsibility would be approaching the friend who knows your struggle and asking them to check in with you once a week, not waiting for them to make the move. Do they know you want this kind of accountability? Are they able? As nice as it would be to have an overachieving and invested friend to check in with you daily without ever been asked, it's not likely going to happen. Accountability takes very intentional conversation. It's up to you to find someone who can commit to that, because not everyone can.

Personal responsibility also involves taking ownership of your behaviours. What do you need to be accountable for? Be clear with yourself and your partner right from the get-go about what behaviours you need support with, and be clear if they change over time.

We must take personal responsibility for our actions. While you may not be responsible for things that happened in the past (e.g. being exposed to porn, abuse or trauma), you are responsible for your recovery in the here and now. Accountability starts with you.

2. *Expectations*

A well-oiled accountability machine doesn't just fall out of the sky. You need to create, work on and maintain it. You do this by being explicit with expectations and putting a game-plan in place. During your first few meet-ups or phone calls as accountability partners, discuss openly some definitive expectations of each other. It can help to even write it down in a 'contract' of sorts, to remind you what you're signing up for.

This is because, as much as we'd like to believe our whole heart is in this, it probably isn't. Why? Because accountability hurts. It's uncomfortable. It means revealing your barest soul to someone and risking rejection. Part of you is always going to want to avoid it. It's way too easy for accountability to fail when you don't have a clear framework.

It's important to begin by getting on the same page as your partner. Are you both ready for the same level of commitment and responsibility? Are your relevant values aligned? If not, try again with someone new. When you find your accountability match, clear and tangible expectations give you the best chance of avoiding 'The Fade'. The Fade is when busyness, awkwardness and reluctant hearts slowly but surely remove us from real accountability. We begin to skip scheduled chats, the hard-hitting questions become vague and it turns into a hang-out session, if we even make it that far. This does our recovery no good. Here, contacting that person in moments of temptation begins to feel 'too bothersome'. We're not sure it matters anymore. It's stopped being intentional. And you're on your way to relapse.

If you want to recover, you must make a plan and both agree to prioritising it. Ask these questions:

- Where will we meet?
- How often will we meet? (I recommend weekly)
- How long will we meet for? (I recommend 1 hour)
- What questions do I need to be asked?
- Will we pray together regularly?
- Is anyone else welcome in this group?
- Will this be confidential?
- What do you need from each other?
- Will your accountability partner be available for emergency texts or calls when you're tempted?
- What are their personal boundaries? Remember, they will not be available 24/7 and you need to be careful of wearing them out.

3. *Consistency*

Fight The Fade with consistency. Regularly meeting together and reviewing your expectations helps to make them a priority. The life of a woman in the 21st Century is busy and chaotic. Whether you're studying, working, living on welfare, or in any other situation, there are many activities and responsibilities that capture our time. However, once you miss one or two meet-ups, it becomes far too easy to continue down this slippery slope. Sometimes, you really can't help missing a week, but always try to stay in touch with your accountability partner somehow in these times. If you're sick, away or stuck at home with a broken-down car, pick up the phone for a quick chat or text an update on how you're really doing. If you don't have reception, email them! If worst comes to worst, you can write a personal journal entry reflecting on the last week's victories or lapses. Although this might be private, it keeps you in a routine of honesty. Shame makes it far too easy to make excuses to avoid accountability. Often the things that make it difficult to be consistent have a legitimate basis, but you need to work with or around them. Don't skip accountability.

4. *Questions*

Questions are vital to accountability and recovery. Our natural tendency is to skimp on real honesty because it's frightening; questions get straight to the point and draw the truth out without prolonging the pain. They can become accountability anchors for honest discussion. Asking and being asked simple, direct questions is one of the best gifts you can give or receive in recovery, even if they make you squirm.

- Have you looked at porn?
- Have you masturbated?

Many women like to use code or euphemisms for these terms to allow discussions to happen honestly in more public places. I've heard women use 'killing kittens' for masturbation and 'having pizza' for porn. I think using the real terms breaks cultural stigma and brings a sense of seriousness and personal responsibility to the conversation, but it's up to you.

The final questions are:

- Why?
- How?

Asking 'why' and 'how' isn't about sharing gory sexual details. Discussing why is about identifying your triggers. You may also like to ask questions such as 'What negative emotion or stress was I feeling the week or day I lapsed?', 'What sexual temptations were available at the time?' or 'What triggered me to seek out porn or sex?'. Alternatively, if you overcame temptation, ask 'What was different this time?', 'What motivated me to resist?' or

'Can I identify anything that made it easier to avoid giving in to temptation?'.

Explaining 'how' includes noting what happened and how you worked around accountability software or other boundaries. This question also applies to celebrating victory! If you resisted temptation, explore what you did to achieve that, and repeat.

Good self-awareness takes time to develop, but will give you the control you need to break free and cut temptation off at the root. Consistently and honestly answering these questions can train you to identify triggers, helpful behaviours and stay on your guard.

5. *Flexibility*

Addiction can make rigid women out of us. It creates a black and white world of good and bad, right and wrong, and we often live in a land of hard and fast rules.

Accountability needs to be structured enough to draw out honest conversation, and consistent enough to be effective, but it must also be flexible. If something isn't working, try something new. If an accountability partner isn't gelling with you, discuss this and if it can't be resolved, find someone new. If phone calls are allowing you too much space to be evasive, meet in person. If sitting in a café makes you panic, try going for a run or chatting over some painting or gardening—whatever activity or setting makes you calm. If your questions are no longer hard-hitting, or you have new recovery needs, discuss this and make changes.

Accountability needs to be intentional and structured, but it doesn't need to be stagnant or rigid. Change is okay. Just ensure you are discussing potential changes with your accountability partner and talk about whether this desire to make change could be an excuse to avoid something scary, like honesty and vulnerability, or if it's a legitimate need.

6. *Positivity*

You're going to discuss struggles and lapses during accountability, but you must also focus on the victories. Celebrate your achievements and share the times you resisted temptation!

My accountability partner and I would organise regular celebratory picnics, bushwalks or gifts for each other to commemorate significant milestones such as three months without a relapse or facing a particularly hairy topic in therapy. These reflect our personalities, but you may prefer other activities; it's all up to you! But I do encourage you to intentionally celebrate and encourage one another on the journey (or, if your partner doesn't struggle ask them to help celebrate and encourage you).

Another way to focus on positivity as you recover is to karate-chop sobriety streak counters out the window. I once used them; I had multiple apps on my phone, and even tried paper trackers and tallies. I loved watching the numbers go up and up and up. I felt like a total bad-ass when I could tell my accountability partners I had over one hundred days of freedom under my belt. It gave a huge sense of achievement and incentive to continue the fight. However, there was a downside.

It was all well and good if my counter was going up daily, but if a lapse did occur, even after two hundred and three days of sobriety, it would reset to a big fat zero and absolutely crush me. I felt like I was right back at the beginning of the journey, on square one yet again. I thought the zero meant I had lost everything I gained over that time, but that wasn't true. There were so many vital aspects to my recovery that were totally ignored by this system of tracking the 'days since'—things like emotional growth, progress in therapy, my ability to keep boundaries, restore intimacy and develop spiritually. I unintentionally oversimplified recovery, a complex and multifaceted journey. Only focusing on one aspect of recovery became another source of shame which I didn't need.

It's important to remember too, that mistakes can be great learning tools. Babies don't learn to walk by making strong declarations of intent and just getting up and wandering away; they gurgle unintelligibly and fall over a thousand times. They eventually learn what works and what doesn't. Falling is an essential part of the learning process. Give yourself the same care and consideration. Failure in recovery is an opportunity to reflect on what you can do better next time.

The solution to failure shame is to implement a slightly different method of tracking. Instead of counting the days since your last slip up (which focuses on a negative), use some kind of marker on a calendar (digital or paper) to track whether you experience a lapse or victory each day. A simple method is to use a red or green dot, but you can create any system you want. You might also want to take note of particular breakthroughs or achieved goals, as well as the not-so-good days. The Fortify Program[2] created by Fight the New Drug is a fantastic recovery program accessed as an app which includes all of these features and many more. This is another great option if you want something that's already set up for you (and free). By honestly tracking your victories and mistakes, you create a much fuller picture of your recovery journey than simply counting how many days since the last screw up. It places emphasis on being honest about your mistakes and the need to push forward in recovery, but also celebrates the positives and urges you to celebrate your personal growth. This is a much more balanced and helpful perspective, especially early on in the journey.

Conclusion

Accountability isn't easy, but it's so, so worth it. Let me finish this chapter with a story. Today, I chatted to my hairdresser about my own journey of installing filtering software, having the reports sent to my best friend, and the gritty reality of accountability. Hairdressers always get the good stuff out of you! I guess it's hard to avoid getting personal when the answer to 'So, what do you do?' is 'I'm writing a book for women struggling with porn.' Anyway, she was shocked and in awe at the lengths I went to in order to overcome my addiction. She was especially horrified and impressed at the thought of my personal browser history being sent to someone! Right now, I stand on the other side of recovery. I don't have to do these radical things anymore, because I gave them my all during my recovery and after every relapse (there were quite a few). Until I heard someone else's exclamation at what I'd done, I had almost forgotten how harrowing the journey of accountability can be. But, let me tell you: it's worth it. You can live in freedom.

I was where you are. You can join me on the glorious podium of recovery too, if you give this your all. Let reality sink in: you truly need accountability. You need someone on your team. You must wisely choose a woman to confide in, speak the truth, install filtering software, implement a plan of action using the six pillars of great accountability and keep at it.

Being honest and letting someone see who you truly are and what you struggle with is one of the most courageous things you can ever do. I know the world tells us courage has to be big and loud and strong, that power comes through force and strength, and making your way through life on your own is noble. But truly, the most courageous, powerful and strong thing you can do is be vulnerable, honest and invite others into your pain. Trust me, if you do the gritty work of being transparent in your recovery, you will inspire others, and one day someone will hear your story and say 'Wow. I can't believe you did that. That took guts!' and it will feel amazing, because you know it's true.

This is the beginning of your restoration.

Action Steps:

1. **Brainstorm a list of women you could approach about accountability.**
2. **Choose one woman, share your struggle with her and ask her to keep you accountable.**
3. **If she agrees, meet up to discuss expectations and details. Ask her to read this chapter.**
4. **Download and install filtering software on all your devices.**

CHAPTER THREE: INVENTORY

In the previous chapter, I mentioned my first experience with accountability through a personal trainer at the gym. It was pretty transformative, not only for my health, but for my understanding of the role of accountability in sexual recovery. I was able to use the values I learned through fitness and adjust them to suit my recovery needs. This experience wouldn't be the last time I'd learn a valuable recovery lesson from the fitness industry. My first trainer taught me the value of accountability, but my second one hit me over the head with the power of inventory.

In standard human fashion, I went hard on the weights and cardio for a good six months and adhered to my accountability obligations with my ridiculously fit trainer. I saw results, but it wasn't long before being comfortable with my routine killed my motivation. A day off here and there became a regular habit, and days turned into weeks without entering that old weight-lifting gym. I stopped taking responsibility for my actions and became comfortable not pushing myself. Life got busy, relationships became complicated and I eventually left the gym to pursue other hobbies—which included stuffing my face with tacos, binging on Netflix and sleeping. I suffered the consequences and ended up back at square one.

After some time, I wandered into a brightly lit women's gym full of shiny weights, machines and ladies clad in overpriced activewear. It was time for something new, I decided. Time for change. Perhaps mixing up my routine would keep me motivated.

Once I'd registered and signed the waiver that I wouldn't sue if I broke my back Zumba-ing too hard, something unexpected happened. Instead of taking my (far too high) membership fee, chucking a 'free' water bottle at me and sending me on my merry way to use the leg press machine backwards, my new fitness mentor asked me to sit with her and avoid working out altogether that very first day. Now this was a gym I could get on board with!

It wasn't a day off though—she had a mental workout in mind. We sat on a comfy lounge and she took my pulse. Not my physical blood flow, but my lifestyle and fitness pulse. Where was I at? What had I tried before? What hadn't worked? Where did I want to be? What does my current lifestyle and diet look like? Did I have any medical conditions? Where was I falling short of my health goals and what could I do about it? She asked me to do small physical tasks such as push ups, squats and vertical leaps to gauge my genuine fitness levels.

Every detail was recorded on a crisp sheet of paper and tucked neatly into the Alice Taylor file. This was my fitness inventory, and I could return to it at any time to remember my goals, get motivated and see the areas that needed special attention. A few months down the track it also served as a great encouragement to see just how far I had come!

Answering personal questions and having them recorded on paper gave me an objective view of reality. Simple but direct questions and tasks revealed both positive and negative habits, and this picture gave me a clear idea of the practical areas to focus on and injected me with a rush of motivation to change. It wasn't all pleasant. In fact, some of it was quite awkward. This task revealed my shortcomings and guilty pleasures and at times I was turning pink from embarrassment. My trainer never shamed me; she was compassionate and kind, but I was certainly uncomfortable (especially when I could only do half a push-up).

I needed this inventory, though. In some areas, I was pleased with my current behaviours. I didn't realise the good I was already doing for my body, but in others I was gobsmacked with how sloppy and unhealthy I had become. This was a lifechanging experience, not only because it supported my goals to improve my strength and health, but because it gave me a guide for my sexual healing. This unassuming health check became the blueprint for a sexual inventory which would set me in good stead for my future. Aside from getting real about how many burgers I was eating a week, it proved to me I needed to get brutally real with myself about how often I was using porn, what other behaviours I was practicing and how it was impacting my everyday relationships and life. That was, if I really wanted to get better.

Enough about gym! What exactly is an inventory?

You may not have participated in a sexual inventory before. It's certainly not something regular people do for fun, but it's important, and a relatively simple recovery tool, if you're a woman struggling with sex.

An inventory of any kind is simply a series of questions relating to your past and current behaviours. In this case, we're talking sexual behaviours. In your head, you probably know you have an issue with porn and masturbation, or random sex and tinder hook-ups. You most likely beat yourself up for this too, because you believe you're the worst of the worst and the only woman struggling. But an inventory can give you a clear and non-judgemental picture of where you are truly at with your struggle. An inventory for recovering women may include questions such as:

- How frequently do you view pornography?
- On a scale of 1-10 how severe would you rate your struggle?
- On a scale of 1-10 how severely would a friend or mentor rate your struggle?
- What consequences have you experienced from your acting out?

Answering these can provide you with a much-needed reality check. The right questions have the power to help you see the truth of your condition, without shame. Inventory can help you gain valuable insight into a number of aspects of your struggle such as:

- The true severity of your struggle.
- Specific acting our behaviours.
- Any success or failures you've had in attempting to get free.
- Why these attempts did or didn't work.
- Other wounded behaviours that need attention.
- The presence of mental illness, trauma or abuse.
- Hidden emotional pain and triggers.
- Relationships or attitudes that keep you trapped in addiction.

It's possible this process may even draw out old memories which have lain dormant for some time; as I walked through an inventory with a friend, I watched her have more than one 'aha!' moment. Answering questions she'd never been asked before helped her connect the dots of her childhood trauma to her current struggles with intimacy and family.

Won't this just make me feel like crap?

Creating a worksheet full of your deepest pain and shame may seem like the most useless activity ever for an already struggling woman—I mean, you already know you have issues, right?! Isn't this just going to make it worse, or confirm the deepest fears you have about yourself? True, there is a legitimate danger that an inventory can send you into a spiral of shame. It may even trigger you to act out as a way to self-soothe the pain. But you never do inventory alone; you do it with the love and support of an accountability partner, friend, mentor or professional. This is your safety net as you deal with potential pain triggers. Not only this, but part of the unique healing power of inventory is in sharing everything with a trusted friend or mentor.

There is nothing more healing than to be fully known and still be loved and accepted. I've officially shared my inventory twice. Once, I filled out a questionnaire from a recovery workbook and handed it over to my mentor. This is a straight-forward method, and gives your accountability partner or counsellor some honest insight into where you're truly at with your struggle. This is a win-win situation, because you get to experience unconditional love and acceptance, and they learn more about how they can support you better. The second time I honestly shared a systematic overview of my life was over Skype a few years later. This inventory was a little different to the basic one included with this guide. Instead of outlining my addictive behaviours and experiences, I listed the things I was most ashamed about—things I had never shared before.

This was an advanced exercise, and I was only able to do it many years after I had stopped using pornography compulsively. It was incredibly healing. As I spoke these secrets out loud to my recovery coach for the first time, I was changed. She validated all my struggles and responded calmly to confessions which I deemed shocking. In this moment, I was able to let go of my shame and remember my worth. You can experience this too. You might like to share your inventory on paper, or you may like to talk through it, discussing particular answers which were meaningful to you. If your accountability partner happens to struggle too, you can talk through your responses together.

I am also adamant that therapy, counselling or mentoring is required to heal from the trauma of addiction—this relationship is a valuable place to share and talk over your inventory answers too. If a specific question triggered a lot for you, therapy is a great place to home in on some of these more tender areas while you continue to move forward in your accountability and sobriety.

It's tough digging up a lifetime of secrets and seeing them on paper, but remember this process isn't intended to shame you. This isn't about using guilt or fear-tactics to alter your behaviour (surely if that worked, you'd be free by now!). With the right support and momentum, your first inventory is actually a life changing and positive activity. An inventory done well will probably bring up feelings of shame and regret, but it is also a place for compassion to be poured out on you. More than this, it will serve as an impetus to really get well.

When you get all your mess out on paper, you can look at it and say 'I no longer want this life.' It can be confronting but following through with the process gives you the ability to move forward. Of course, healing from a lifetime of pain takes time; it won't be immediate, and you'll need to invest in therapy and recovery work, but an honest, physical inventory is the beginning of leaving the junk behind you. You have moved the tangle of emotions and experiences from your mind and put them on paper. These are hard truths, but stripping them of secrecy also removes their power. Naming the experiences of the past gives you an opportunity to look to the future, to take on the next day unencumbered by the secrets of the past. Imagine dealing with just one day's troubles, instead of being burdened by every other day of your life as well.

Inventory is about taking your power back. It's about letting go of all deception, denial and excuses so you can begin to take responsibility for your current life and behaviours. It's a tool that empowers you to look into the future and decide what you want from life. It's a practice in courage and integrity with the power to catapult you into a life of wholeness and healing.

The bulk of this chapter comes in worksheet form. Instead of reading my words, you'll be filling out your own! This is your chance to make this guide yours, and start taking action for your recovery, rather than sitting on the sidelines reading about it. Before you download your sexual inventory from The Grace Spot, there's another side to inventory that you need to understand. Just as important as examining your unwanted behaviours is tracking your attitude towards, and participation in, self-care. Attending to your basic needs is vital to your healing, and another behaviour to record on paper.

Self-care Tracker

Let's talk about tracking your basic needs and self-care behaviours. Recovery is about identifying and eliminating unwanted behaviours, but it is not only about removing things from your life. It is also about restoration! If self-care, love and the provision of your basic human needs are lacking, they must be restored to your life in order to fully heal.

Think of a proud sunflower. Its petals and leaves become infected and die off. The gardener sees this, and responds by pruning it back and removing the dead or sickly parts. But now it's just a tall green stick in the dirt. The clued-in gardener knows to nurture the soil in order to bring that beauty back to life. What does the plant need? Sunlight, water, fertiliser, protection from insects or birds and, some might even say, song to help them grow taller. When the plant is cared for, and its basic needs are met, it flourishes. It is restored to its former glory and more. You are the sunflower, bright and beautiful. Yes, there will be pruning and restriction, but you were created to flourish and shine, not just have your 'dead parts' chopped off. Self-care is part of how we do this.

We share a need for sunlight, water and care with the sunflower, but I've created a list of basic human needs the woman in recovery should be aware of that the sunflower may not be so keen on. There are six categories: Physical, relational, spiritual, restorative, sobriety and emotional. You are welcome to add your own customised headings and dot points, but I find these touch on most women's needs in recovery, and you'll want to avoid overcomplicating it.

Physical

- Healthful eating and drinking
- Adequate sleep and rest
- Attending to medical and hygienic needs
- Joyful movement
- Practicing body kindness

Getting adequate sleep, exercise, nutrition and avoiding negative self-talk all have a positive effect on your overall health and wellbeing, which in turn will help you continue to live in freedom. The better you feel, the less likely you are to turn to porn. You don't need to become a health junkie to improve your wellbeing, but it's helpful to reflect on any imbalances in this area. Food restriction (i.e. extreme dieting) or binge eating (including comfort eating), focusing on parts of your body you don't like, and placing moral judgement on different types of food (e.g. kale is 'good' and chocolate is 'bad') are all unhelpful habits. Healthful eating leaves you satisfied, not feeling sick or starving, and includes mostly nutritious foods—but certainly not exclusively. Sometimes, cake is self-care too! The same goes for exercise: both a sedentary life and excessive training can damage you mentally and physically. Seek balance and listen to your body's needs, rather than stressing out trying to change or punish it. This is the crux of physical self-care. You can find inspiration to pursue great self-care in *Body Positive Power*[1] and *Health at Every Size*[2].

Relational

- Connecting with safe and loving people, practicing non-sexual intimacy
- Present with children (if applicable)
- Pursuing harmony, peace and unity with intimate partner (if applicable)

Spiritual

- Practicing spiritual disciplines (e.g regular prayer)
- Feeling connection with God and fellow believers

A woman's personal faith and church community can be an incredible source of joy and encouragement; however, we must acknowledge that church also has the capacity to become a ripe breeding ground for shame; many women have already experienced this. Spiritual disciplines and activities such as attending church, volunteering, giving financially or serving in ministry can become guilt practices. Many Christian women try to 'make up' for their sins by serving more or drowning themselves in 'duties' like Bible reading or church cleaning. Beware of the intention behind your spiritual practices. Are they stemming from guilt or shame? Do they burden you further? If so, they are not restorative or helpful for your spiritual healing. Spiritual self-care may look like stepping back from some of these pressures, and exploring alternative practices to help you connect with God and your spiritual community.

Restorative practices

- Participating in a hobby, sport or activity that is unrelated to work or recovery
- Avoiding excessive screen time

Just as porn addiction and shame can be consuming; so too can recovery. Whether you're constantly thinking about pornography—or focusing all your energy on not using it—it remains the central focus of your life. This is why it is so important to invest in hobbies, projects or activities that are totally unrelated to recovery. Give your body and mind a break from the mental load of working through your issues. Do something that makes you feel alive, that refreshes you. There's more to your life than either watching porn or trying not to watch porn. Plus, spending a tonne of time staring at a screen will only make you feel like trash.

Sobriety

- Checking in with accountability partner
- Abstaining from acting out behaviours
- Avoiding substitutes for sexually acting out and obsessive behavior.
- Attending counselling, therapy or mentoring

Emotional

- Aware of emotions and managing them well
- Generally content and optimistic about the future

It's okay to feel sad, angry, afraid or other unpleasant emotions. This isn't about pretending to be happy when you're not, but rather being mindful and reflective of your emotions, being honest with yourself and others about them and taking precautions to avoid becoming overwhelmed. This may include journaling, art or another creative outlet, debriefing with a friend or mentor or just being able to mindfully identify what you're feeling, and why. Avoid suppressing your emotions or attempting to medicate negative ones with unhelpful behaviours.

Self-care leads the way to healing

Attending to these basic needs are the foundation upon which growth and self-actualisation occurs. Without a strong foundation of self-care it will be difficult to recover well and be a functional woman working on healing. Intentionality and responsibility when it comes to self-care are part of restoration. It's just as important as leaving behind negative behaviours, and will bolster your healing journey. Self-care is a super power you give yourself.

Assessing your ongoing self-care habits can provide tremendous insight into your recovery. You may realise there are areas in which you are consistently missing the mark (too much screen time, not enough sleep anyone?). This may be a vital piece of the recovery puzzle that's been holding you back for years. Just like the sexual addiction inventory, tracking your self-care habits helps you identify patterns and improve your life moving forward. In our busy lives, especially as women, attending to our basic physical and emotional needs often gets pushed aside for others. We miss out. It feels like the easiest sacrifice in your week full of appointments, meetings, childminding and engaging with your world. In fact, you may not even notice you're doing it. Yet, letting self-care fall by the wayside has a huge impact on your ability to function well in all those other settings you're prioritising, particularly when it comes to relationships. Engaging with self-care, and tracking your attempts, will improve your recovery. You've got to fill your tank, girl!

Once you've completed this chapter, download the self-care tracker from The Grace Spot. You'll find directions on how to do so in the Action Steps at the end of the chapter. Put it somewhere accessible and easily seen and track your activities for six weeks. You may be surprised how little time you give to nurturing yourself or participating in restful and lifegiving activities. Recovery is about sobriety and restoration. You can't find freedom without practicing both. Continue using the tracker (just download another one for free) if you find it helpful, and remember: you're not striving for perfection. No one ever gets it right. This is simply a useful tool to gauge where you sit on the spectrum of self-care, and if you need to dedicate more time to it. This is not about the numbers, it's about self-reflection and awareness. Trust me, you'll never get your ten out of ten on this one because life is crazy! This is simply a reminder to do your best when you can.

Conclusion

Doing an inventory of any kind is a courageous practice in reflection and honesty. It is an opportunity rarely encountered in our modern culture, so even though it's uncomfortable and feels way too vulnerable, this is a chance to jump fully on board and experience all this process has to offer. As you catalogue your past experiences and evaluate your current life in terms of dysfunctional sexual behaviour and the ability to put yourself in the way of self-care, you are giving yourself the gift of hindsight and motivation. An honest inventory will not only help you understand the journey you've been on and identify problem areas, but it stands to be a motivator for change in your life.

This is a rare opportunity to lay down your defences, excuses, justifications and that nasty pointing finger that shrugs responsibility onto an outside source, and finally speak honestly to yourself and a trusted person. Integrity may feel like an unfamiliar trait in your world of sexual struggle and cover-ups. It may feel unachievable and frightening—but you're already on your way to a life of true integrity. By honestly admitting your condition, seeking accountability and now, practicing a fearless inventory, you are starting something new. You are healing. You are becoming the woman you truly are inside. You're being restored, and creating a rock-solid foundation on which to leap off into the future.

Now you've read through this explanation of what inventory is, and how to practice it, you're ready to head over to The Grace Spot and download both the self-care tracker and the sexual addiction inventory. You can find these listed under 'Get Help' followed by 'Download Worksheets' which you'll find in the 'Read my Book' section or at thegracespot.com/Restored-worksheets.

These downloads are free, and you are able to access them for an unlimited time, as many times as you need.

Action Steps:

1. **Download the sexual addiction inventory and self-care tracker from The Grace Spot.**
2. **Print these out and fill them in.**
3. **Once you've completed these, share them with a trusted friend, accountability partner, therapist or mentor. Discuss standout questions and answers.**

CHAPTER FOUR: THE MASTURBATION CONTROVERSY

Welcome. We've arrived at a topic which is possibly even more taboo than women and pornography. It's time to discuss The-M-Word. Touching yourself. Fapping. Self-stimulation. Jacking off. Jilling off. Pushing the love button. Ringing Satan's doorbell. That thing. Doin' it. Pants-down-time. Happy time. Special time. Tickling the hairy oyster. Killing kittens. Solo sex. Onan's curse.

Masturbation.

Whatever you want to call it, it's a polarising topic in the Christian world. And the debate can get heated. Unfortunately, these theological and moral debates haven't achieved much in the way of helping women actually heal from addiction. Neither has the echoing silence that characterises many church communities. These have only served to create a deeper sense of shame as women are either told outright they are wrong for masturbating, or it is treated like women and porn: no one is doing it, and if they are, it's too bad to talk about. Where rigid opinions and debate intersect with private sexuality, shame thrives, and women are given even more reason to remain silent and isolated.

The purpose of the following discussion isn't to discover the 'right answer' or tick 'solve the masturbation debate' off our to-do list. This is not simply a theological or moral investigation either (I've found these tend to skimp out on reality), but a place to freely consider whether masturbation is in fact a helpful or unhelpful behaviour in your personal recovery. This is your recovery; you get to choose what it looks like. You get to decide what behaviours work and don't work for you, and how you address them. Then, you can take your conviction and be clear about it with yourself, and your accountability partner. Trust me, if you don't decide now, it is far too easy to use that lack of clarity to become secretive and to start masturbating all the way down that slippery slope of addiction.

Most women in recovery know from the get-go that masturbation is either a top line (acceptable) or bottom line (unacceptable) behaviour for them. I've seen it first-hand. There's something in some women's guts that just shouts 'No! you can't do this, girl!', while others genuinely recover better by allowing it. As much as we Christians hate it, this is another one of those grey areas with no simple answer. It's personal, complex and important. This means there are also a lot of women who are confused and have no idea whether they should be restricting or not. So, we need to talk about it.

No excuses

This discussion is not an invitation to let your wildest and mildest excuses run free. I deliberated over publishing this chapter for fear that women of conviction may read stories of other women who allow masturbation, and get caught up in desire. I worried that justification may slip into this discussion, leading recovering women to relapse. I know just how easy it is for excuses to form in the privacy and isolation of our own minds. They can become scarily convincing. But this isn't about comparison. This isn't about taking what works for one woman and exploiting her story to fit your own justifications for wounded behaviours.

Rather, this chapter is a gift. It is an opportunity to be responsible for your own healing, to be honest and practice using your integrity. As you read through stories, opinions and facts, it is a chance to grow in wisdom and freedom. This is your chance to courageously and honestly examine yourself, your beliefs, values and experiences and to stand up for what you know is true in your heart. This is your opportunity to pull back your favourite excuses and dig deep into the part of you that knows what is going to be genuinely helpful or unhelpful for your lasting recovery and restoration.

No one else can dictate your recovery; in order to heal well you must get in tune with your own heart. You need to throw off judgement and face the topic with a level and determined head. So, let's get to it.

The following chapter allows you to examine the masturbation debate without all the judgement and shame you may be used to. In it, we will discuss:

1. The heart behind the desire.
2. Is masturbation sinful or not?
3. Outside of spiritual morality, what are the pros to masturbation?
4. Outside of spiritual morality, what are the cons of masturbation?

But first, before we begin to delve into the information, let me acknowledge the women who struggle exclusively with masturbation, who have never been addicted to pornography. Your struggle is real and valid, and I believe applying the principals in this book will be helpful for your recovery. However, this chapter is directed towards women who struggle with pornography primarily, who also masturbate. Be mindful as you read this chapter that it may be triggering, and to read with caution, understanding that the advice given may not be helpful to your specific struggle.

The heart behind the desire

When the controversial topic of masturbation comes up at events I'm speaking at, I am bombarded with questions and opinions. Women are absolutely desperate to know if masturbation is acceptable. They want to know if what they've probably all been doing is 'okay'.

'Is it sinful?'

'What if I can do it without lust?'

'Does Jesus condemn masturbation?'

'Is it healthy?'

'Should I masturbate before getting married?'

'Is masturbation within marriage okay?'

'Will legions of demons set up camp in my hoo-haa if I get busy down there?'

I'll be honest with you; I am going to deconstruct the debate and address many of these queries so you can make an informed decision ... but these are all the wrong questions! I've found that asking whether masturbation is sinful or not can really become a detour around the real issue...which is your heart. In other words, what is your motivation? Why are you so invested in this discussion in the first place? I believe answering these questions takes priority over trying to figure out the morality of the behavior.

It's important to identify your motivation before we move on to more concrete ideas surrounding the morality of masturbation and its place in the Christian woman's life. Know your heart, ladies! It can be a slippery sucker. Always wanting what it wants without the slightest worry of logic or consequences. Rules and regulations can be manipulated. They become a wall, begging to be climbed or knocked down. I believe it is far more valuable to establish your motivation first. When conviction comes from the heart it sticks.

What is your motivation?

When it comes to masturbation, do you feel like you need it to be okay? Are you desperately searching for a loophole? Do you feel you need masturbation because:

- You worry you will never experience sex/intimacy with someone?
- It is the only relief you can get from emotional or physical stress?
- It is your only comfort when you feel down?
- It is a way to escape reality for a while?
- You physically can't stop?
- You worry what you would do if you couldn't do it?

If you answered yes to any of these questions, this may indicate masturbation is actually a core part of your addiction. This may indicate an underlying dependence on masturbation to disengage from reality, which means it isn't simply a physical practice but an act which represses emotions and healing. Even if the 'rules' which will follow end up saying 'it's okay to masturbate', it may be wise to remain abstinent from it anyway.

Some more helpful questions to ask of yourself are these:

- Why am I so invested in this debate?
- Am I motivated by fear, shame and rigidity?
- Am I in touch with my motivation and emotions?
- Why does this topic make me feel the way it does?
- If someone forbade me to masturbate, how would I react? Why?
- If someone gave me the green light, how would I react? Why?
- What people or events have coloured my views of masturbation and sexuality?

Of course, with a topic so controversial, personal, sexual, circumstantial and especially with addiction and relgion tied into it, it's likely you're uncertain about it all. It's understandable if your heart is twisted around the 'yes', the 'no', and the plain confused. It's okay if you don't really know the answer to the earlier questions yet. No one ever truly sits in the black and white.

The compulsion and draw towards masturbation can be the result of trauma, abuse, abandonment, neglect and loneliness. Sometimes it's simply our sex drive saying 'Hello world!'. Masturbation doesn't always mean your heart is a mess, it can just mean your heart is beating fast because you're turned on, like any other woman in the world.

Before you put all your hopes and desires into the discussion for or against touching yourself, consider exposing and exploring your heart, first. This way, even if the Scriptures and 'authorities' on sex turn out to say 'yes, masturbate all day, every day, with no consequences!', you can rest assured in a conviction that comes from your heart.

Is masturbation sinful or not?

Let's get to those more practical questions then, shall we? Probably the most common query from Christian women on this topic is 'is masturbation sinful?'. The best place to find answers to spiritual ponderings such as these is the Bible, of course. Here's what it says about women and masturbation…

Nothing. Nada. Blank.

Unfortunately, it's difficult to get a clear picture of what God thinks of masturbation because the Bible doesn't address it specifically. But don't worry, that's not an excuse to throw caution to the wind and masturbate your way through life. There are clues throughout the Scriptures which we can use to figure out what God thinks. There are passages and stories which relate to similar topics, which give us some insight.

The sin of Onan

Genesis 38:8-10

Some Christians believe this passage clearly condemns masturbation. If you aren't familiar with this text, basically a dude named Onan is having sex with a woman named Tamar (his sister-in-law, to be exact) but 'spills his seed'. And no, he didn't knock over the pot plant on the bedside table; he pulled out, and his sperm didn't make it to the egg. In the text, God condemns Onan for this act and punishes him by death (yikes). Some have interpreted this as condemning masturbation, as for men a similar 'spilling' occurs, without the purpose of procreation. However, this feels like a weak link to me. It seems that Onan was clearly directed to impregnate Tamar in order to raise up an heir after her husband died, as was required by Jewish law. By pulling out, he directly disobeyed God. I believe it is his disobedient heart and actions that are condemned, not his wasted sperm. You're welcome to investigate this further but, to my eyes, this seems a poor substitute for a biblical foundation against masturbation (and the pulling-out method, if you're wondering).

The Sermon on the Mount

Matthew 5:27-29

By far the most significant thing the Bible has to say on the topic is in Jesus' sermon recorded in Matthew. Among other things, he discusses the topic of lust. While not specifically about women touching their bits, we can make the connection, right? Let's be honest, most midnight- masturbation-marathons involve at least a little (okay, I mean a lot) of sexual fantasy and lust.

Jesus says thinking lustful thoughts are morally equal to acting them out. As a Christian, are you open to pre-marital sex, adultery, or sexual activity outside of a monogamous marriage? Would you do these things in reality? It seems Jesus is saying, if you see an issue with these active behaviours, you should be taking issue with the fantasies in your mind, too. God looks at the condition of your heart, and what's in your mind, not simply your behaviours.

Jesus places serious weight on lust. He even says if your right eye causes you to sin, pluck it out! If your arm causes you to sin, chop it off and throw it away! I'm going to go out on a *limb* here and say that's a hyperbole, because alongside His other teachings, self-mutilation doesn't really fit. I believe He's simply emphasising that sin, including lust, has devastating consequences and should be avoided.

It seems pretty clear that lust is a no-no for the Christian woman of integrity. If you want to obey Jesus, it's best to steer clear (I know, it's frustrating, isn't it?). Which brings us to our next question—the one that always seems to come next …

What if I do it without lust?

While not always the case, it sure looks like you're Olympic diving through some loopholes here. Is your heart fighting for a way to stay in your masturbatory ways? This is a great time to check in with yourself and the motivation behind your questions. Are you genuinely curious, or are you desperate for some kind of loophole? For the curious and thoughtful, some brave women have shared their experiences with masturbation for this book to help us think through the topic.

Su Lee struggled with compulsive pornography use, sex and fantasy for many years. Masturbation was certainly part of this. When she began her recovery journey, she discussed her top/bottom line behaviours with her therapist and accountability partner. She decided that porn, sex and sexual fantasy were off limits. She wanted to cull these behaviours from her life, and took steps to do so. As a Christian, she agreed with the biblical mandate to flee lustful thoughts and actions. She knew this included masturbating to fantasies, even if the men weren't real people she knew. However, she believes on occasion, she is able to masturbate without lust, and this helps to quieten her craving for porn and sex. She is honest with her accountability partner and therapist about when and how often she masturbates, and if fantasy or porn slip into the practice. She has cut some behaviours out entirely, and left masturbation—but it's important to note it's masturbation with boundaries and accountability. It's not reckless and unnamed. And she remains open to re-evaluating.

Su Lee's story is just one example of a Christian woman continuing to engage with the act of masturbation during her recovery. Adelaide is another woman who shared her story with me, through Facebook. She also participates in lust free masturbation and believes the instructions on freedom, thankfulness and glorifying God in relation to 'unclean' food in 1 Corinthians 10 can be translated to participating in masturbation. One must be thankful to God and focused on glorifying Him through the sexual act, as a married couple might do through intercourse.

What do you think about lust free masturbation?

Do you think it's possible? It's certainly debatable. Personally, I've tried it. It's not easy. It's tough to keep a blank mind, or focus on something totally asexual, on the road to orgasm! I do think it's possible, just difficult. In the end it's up to you to know what's possible and helpful for you. Is it something you can keep up with? Or are you concerned you'll slip into fantasy and need more visual stimulation? This has certainly been a familiar story over the years as I've walked with women in recovery. It takes a strong will to close off your mind to sexual thoughts while masturbating, and I've known a number of women who have started out allowing the act to remain in their lives, but who have experienced a full-blown relapse.

Some simply swapped out porn with masturbation, and continued to live in addictive behaviours, ignoring their negative emotions. Others did well for a long time but eventually relaxed their boundaries and found themselves in fantasy-land again, either in their mind or through a screen.

Wisdom says, if lust free masturbation is to be part of your journey, it isn't a free for all. To give yourself the best chance at recovering long-term, it is important to have boundaries, support and to be continually reflecting on the state of your life and behaviours, and be willing to change if necessary. Su Lee is a great example of this; she allows masturbation, but with strict boundaries to stay on top of her emotional and spiritual wellbeing.

God's glory (not morning glory)

There's probably a lot more that could be said on the biblical masturbation debate. I think endless books could be written from both perspectives, and they'd probably use the same Bible passages to defend their different opinions. But for now, I hope I've shared enough of both sides of the discussion to get you really thinking about what's best for you. To finish the discussion on the spiritual morality of masturbation, I'd like to leave you with two passages from the New Testament that have stimulated deep conviction and reflection within myself on my own journey. They don't need much explanation, simply an open heart willing to be honest about what it brings up within you.

'I have the right to do anything,' you say—but not everything is beneficial. 'I have the right to do anything'—but not everything is constructive. No one should seek their own good, but the good of others. 1 Corinthians 10:23-24

So whether you eat or drink or whatever you do, do it all for the glory of God. Do not cause anyone to stumble, whether Jews, Greeks or the church of God— even as I try to please everyone in every way. For I am not seeking my own good but the good of many, so that they may be saved. 1 Corinthians 10: 31-33

It appears that lust, at least, is a no-go from a biblical perspective. But let's look beyond the Bible for a moment (don't worry, my conservative friends—Jesus is still here with us). I do believe Scripture is essential for our daily (and eternal) lives, but I also know that reality is complex and there are things the Bible simply doesn't address. We can't only think theologically about our existence; human nature is messy and complicated. There's more to it than just 'it's a sin' or 'it's not a sin'. There are ways that masturbation can affect women both positively and negatively, that we should discuss.

Outside of spiritual morality, what are the pros to masturbation?

Masturbation may be useful as 'sexual methadone'.

You've probably heard that porn is like a drug. It affects your brain in the same way heroin or cocaine can. Both behaviour and substance can become addictive, and users may become dependent, requiring heavier doses to experience the chemical 'rush' (more on this in chapter five). With both sexual behaviours and drug use, withdrawals are a common struggle when beginning the recovery journey. They may be physical or emotional. Life without escapism is a whole new world for the addict and sometimes just dealing with the emotions that used to be managed by their behaviour is enough to send them back to their addiction.

The solution for heroin or other opioid addicts is a little something called methadone. It is a prescription drug which eases difficult withdrawal symptoms to make the transition to sobriety possible in those first few weeks or months. It is a controlled and safer substance, but is still addictive in itself and carries risk. It has been used successfully to treat recovering addicts and is a widely accepted method.

The sex or porn addict, on the other hand, is expected to make a full recovery by going 'cold turkey' overnight.

Assuming they are unmarried, the addict is encouraged to remove every sexual outlet in their life. Why do we expect success if we know other addictions are so difficult to recover from without a pseudo-drug, or at least a gradual weaning process?

What if instead of eliminating absolutely everything—which, much like a starvation diet, encourages relapse or bingeing—the addict could work on individual struggles one at a time? Masturbation may be the final frontier to conquer. What if it helped them to truly find freedom?

Perhaps masturbation could be methadone for the recovering sex addict.

Yet, I see how apt humans are at abusing what is given to us. Our sinful natures propel us to exploit even what is pure, let alone things that sit in the grey area. Is there a way this could actually work in reality? Perhaps it is simply an idealistic theory, or maybe it's exactly what we need to find some balance, but I'll let each individual work that out for herself.

Masturbation without shame might decrease temptation.

What if shame and restriction were the real issue here, rather than the act of masturbation itself?

The shame you feel isolates you, feeding your mind damaging lies. It tells you, 'you are unworthy, you are unlovable!', defying the words God speaks over you. Shame hides you from community and hinders relationships. It acts as a nebulous gap between yourself and your saviour, Jesus. You may place the emphasis of these damages on masturbation. While the act itself can damage and harm relationships, I would say it is not those few moments under your blankets at night that hurt you most. Rather, it is the shame that haunts you every hour. It is constant, and heightened in the wake of a 'slip up'. As you will see in the next chapter, shame or woundedness are the foundation upon which addiction thrives. It is the starting point of the addiction cycle—which is why porn is so hard to beat. You feel shame, use porn to escape that shame, then feel even more shame after that. The cycle goes on.

Imagine if you were able to give that shame the boot, if you stopped giving it so much weight in your life. What if failure didn't rule your heart and identity? I think many women who struggle with masturbation would begin to experience freedom.

What if masturbation wasn't a forbidden behaviour? I've been researching intuitive eating recently, especially for children. I think it's a wonderful way of life to increase wellness, but it's also a great analogy for this topic, too.

The basic theory behind intuitive eating is this: diets don't work, because restriction leads to binging. It's just how our bodies work; they were created to survive during famine. To your body, a diet or restricting a major food group (why do women fight carbs so hard?!) feels like famine, and it responds accordingly by upping your hunger cues and encouraging you to eat like crazy when you can. Think about little kids who are forbidden to eat lollies; when they find them, they lose it and make themselves sick. Eating intuitively, by listening to your hunger and satiety cues and eating whatever food you want without restriction is the solution. In the absence of restriction, your body relaxes and responds to food in a healthy way. If both children and adults are allowed to eat treats sometimes, they won't feel the need to down an entire ice-cream cake on their own at midnight, because they know that tasty food is always available. They don't need to save it up for the 'famine' or have one last hurrah before never eating chocolate again, and it works! It takes time to adjust, and to learn to understand your body's hunger cues, but intuitive eating can effectively combat the cycle of restriction and binging and help you experience genuine satisfaction so you can live the rest of your life well.

I think it could be possible to use this concept when discussing masturbation. Restriction can make things more desirable, exciting and enticing. There's a thrill about gaining access to something previously off-limits. Forbidden behaviours or activities create curiosity, and often, obsession. Think about when you were a teenager—didn't you just want to do everything your parents forbade? Restriction without non-judgemental discussion and reasoning creates a shroud of mystery that the more rebellious amongst us will seek to uncover. I wonder if, like a child restricted of sweet treats, we as grown women become obsessed with masturbation and fantasy simply because it is so intensely restricted and shamed. I don't think this is because we're rebellious or 'bad', it's simply an act that has been unintentionally raised up on a pedestal and given much more power than it should have. I wonder if, like teenagers given permission to do once-forbidden activities (such as skipping church, trying Mum and Dad's alcohol, etc.), women could partake in masturbation without shame or limit, and actually dampen their desire for it. If women know they're allowed to masturbate when they want, if they're not worried it's going to be the 'last time', if it's not something obsessed about or covered in shame … maybe the desire will just eliminate itself. Perhaps, like intuitive eating, masturbation without the shame or restriction could lead to genuine satisfaction, allowing women to live the rest of their lives uninterrupted by the constant desire for orgasm.

Masturbating freely might be the thing that frees you from masturbation.

Masturbation as sex therapy.

As well as those struggling with compulsive sexual behaviours, it is necessary to consider another group of people. Unfortunately, often forgotten in the Christian conversation on self-stimulation are women with sexual dysfunction.

Consider the married woman who has been terribly abused in her past. Now, any sexual touch triggers an inability to have intercourse. Vaginismus is a common issue for women, which causes a great deal of distress and pain. There are many factors contributing to issues such as this, and many more ways it can manifest.

It is wise to invest in sex therapy or counselling for these issues. Often, therapists will suggest gradual masturbation as part of the healing process. Doing this can overcome physical limitations as well as empowering a survivor to reclaim pleasure or sexuality. It may be the only way for a couple to participate in intercourse, which is a sacred and holy part of marriage.

When someone stands out the front of church and condemns masturbation and those who participate in it without considering the complexities or exceptions, more people get hurt. This may become a barrier to both their personal healing, and relationship with God. We must not forget these people.

Masturbation may be what God uses to heal them.

Outside of spiritual morality, what are the cons of masturbation?

Regular masturbation can negatively affect marital sex.

Many people claim that it's important to know your own body before getting married and having sex; masturbation is viewed as 'training' or 'preparation' for the honeymoon. Once you know what you like, you can teach your partner and live orgasmically ever after.

I totally see where these folks are coming from. Going from zero to sixty on your wedding night is kind of intense, and I'm sure there have been women (and men) whose intimate relationship has been made easier by masturbatory experience. I'm not denying that, but my own experience was completely different. And I'm not alone. I want to share a warning with you as you decide whether to embrace, restrict or moderate the act of masturbation in your life.

Mine and Lukas' wedding day was a beautiful blur. We woke up way too early in our separate beds in different houses, said our vows, paid too much for everything, and had an amazing time eating a pink fairy floss pavlova wedding cake (yes, that happened!). We tolerated the photos and festivities, but when the night closed, we literally ran out of the reception hall and punched our hotel address into Google Maps. We were going to have actual sex! Finally!

That first time was special. However, over the course of the honeymoon, we found something wasn't quite right. Sex was disappointing, frustrating and not nearly as orgasmic as we both expected. We realised our histories with masturbation had negatively impacted our sex life.

Masturbation had taught us to expect great sex and great orgasms every time. After ten or so years of consistent masturbation, whether that was accompanied by porn, fantasy or lust free thoughts. It was quick, pleasurable and consistent. It was often an escape from the discomforts of life. It was reliably good. Of course, when it came to real sex, we expected the same thing.

Effectively, pleasuring ourselves, along with the influence of Hollywood, modern culture and porn, taught us sex would be easy. Every encounter would result in great sex and great orgasms, for both of us … every time. Wasn't it supposed to be like super-charged masturbation?

We were both ready for the fireworks show. Alas, it never came. Masturbation taught our bodies to respond to one thing only. It was not for lack of love, affection or effort that our intimacy struggled on the honeymoon. It was our bodies listening to what we'd taught them.

We had both set ourselves up for specific stimulation, in a specific time frame. It was all about 'my pleasure' in 'my time'. By virtue, I could never please him like he'd learned for ten years. And likewise, him for me. Sex is different when there's two of you. Our hands and bodies felt different, they worked differently, and moved differently. We had access to body parts foreign to us until we said our vows. It was entirely different to self-stimulation. And in many cases, not as good. Whatever we were doing to each other, it just didn't feel right.

We were like two Atlantic salmon flailing about on top of each other, trying to find the right spot. We gave up many times, exhausted and pretty damn disappointed. It was frustrating that we'd both accustomed our bodies to respond to XYZ and the other was doing ABC. It was worse than trying to direct someone to scratch an itch on your back, in juuust the right spot. There is not much more dangerous for intimacy than thinking 'I can do this better' when your spouse is trying to serve you.

The result of this was confusion and disappointment. I began to wonder if there was something wrong with me. I questioned why he didn't want to have sex *all the time,* and why he didn't seem to love it when we did. We were both disillusioned with sex, and frustrated that our expectations turned out to be so wrong.

As doom and gloom as this all sounds, let me remind you that *everyone* brings baggage to the marriage bed. Masturbation issues aren't especially heinous, dangerous or shameful. It's just one thing out of many that can impact sex. The beauty of marriage is the covenant of unconditional love, in which all struggles and issues can be resolved and worked through in love. My husband and I, together with prayer and the help of our pre-marriage counsellors, were able to work through our issues, and truly it brought us closer together and created an intimate bond. Plus, our sex life has definitely improved—a lot.

What I learned in those first few weeks of marriage was that when you masturbate, you take your spouse (or future spouse) out of the equation. I don't think masturbating in singleness is going to doom your sex life, but be aware it may cause complications, especially in the beginning.

Masturbation doesn't increase self-control.

If you can't say no to yourself when you're alone, you're setting up a poor precedent for your dating and engaged life. By acting on the sexual urge every time it randomly pops in to say hi, you become obedient to it.

What will stop you from being obedient to that craving when the possibility of real-life intimacy is available?

You should also consider the fact that marriage won't satisfy your every sexual craving. There will be times when one spouse is sexually unavailable for any number of reasons, so wisdom tells me it is good to come to terms with this reality now, and practice self-control, rather than normalising instant gratification whenever your body demands sex. Let us learn to live with integrity and wisdom now, in order to better serve and love our potential future spouses. Look at quitting masturbation as training for the reality of two humans coming together.

Masturbation can become addictive.

Masturbation can be addictive. There's no question about it—people can become dependent on the act, and that is not healthy. It can become an unhelpful coping mechanism, and sabotage good emotional regulation and health. The way to identify if masturbation has become unhelpful for you is to ask these few questions and be honest with yourself:

1. Am I using masturbation to alter my mood?

If you're regularly masturbating in response to negative emotion, you might have a problem. It can indicate you're living in some level of distress, which makes it the perfect opportunity to get hooked—addiction loves pain. If you continually escape reality, and refuse to face your struggles head-on, you won't end up in a place of happiness, and you might not fully recover.

2. Do I feel like I can't stop?

Perhaps one of the clearest signs of addiction is when you feel like you can't stop, even when you really want to. Do you really want to be a slave to your desires? Perhaps it's time to assert some control and make a change.

3. Is my habit harming me or those around me?

Harm can come in many forms: emotional, relational, physical, spiritual or criminal to name a few. If you become so focused on pleasuring yourself whenever you desire that you become isolated and start putting your own pleasure before others' needs, I would suggest masturbation has too much weight in your life.

4. Is my masturbation SAFE?

Dr Patrick Carnes advises his patients to regularly assess if their behaviours are SAFE: S-secretive, A-abusive, F-feelings (mood altering), E-empty (of care and relationship)[1]. If any behaviour falls into any of these categories, it poses a risk to the persons recovery and safety and should be re-evaluated.

Eliza's story

Earlier, Su Lee shared her personal experience of being pro-masturbation. To finish this discussion, I thought I should share one more story from an alternative perspective. Eliza contacted me after hearing me speak at a conference and generously shared her story and gave permission for it to be shared in this chapter.

Eliza is adamant masturbation has no place in her life whatsoever. After struggling with addictive behaviours including pornography, masturbation, chronic fantasy and cybersex with strangers, she cannot separate the behaviours. She knows allowing herself to masturbate would hinder her recovery and possibly even lead to a relapse. She understands the slippery slope that comes with allowing one behaviour to remain, when it has historically been so associated with other acting out behaviours which she is trying to eliminate and heal from. Since she hit rock bottom and realised she needed to recover and seek out a new life, it has always been clear to her that masturbation is a symptom of her addiction, and doesn't help her recovery—even though she quietly wishes she could keep it. However, with her accountability partner, she is honest and seeks to avoid masturbation, with or without fantasy, at all costs. She believes this will lead her into a new life, and full recovery.

Conclusion

This has been a controversial discussion, but I dearly hope it has opened your heart to non-judgemental and genuine consideration. The aim of this chapter was to deconstruct the debate and open a safe space for you to start practicing your integrity and courage. This was an opportunity to be responsible for yourself and your own recovery, a chance for you to be empowered in your convictions, as you hold all options freely.

Starting with prayer for wisdom, give yourself time to re-read this chapter, do further research and mull over the topic. Then ask yourself, 'Should masturbation have a place in my recovery?'. Listen to your gut reaction, what does it say? Catch your initial response to the question before justification, shame or other voices interrupt. It may not be what you want or like, but that little voice is probably integrity speaking. Listen to it.

This choice may only be for a season. I have changed my opinion on masturbation a number of times as new seasons and people taught me new perspectives, and as I matured in self-awareness and listened to stories from amazing women who believed and lived differently to me. Allow yourself the flexibility to change during your recovery, but do so with the support and input of an accountability partner—and always with prayer.

Action Steps:

1. **Pray for wisdom as you decide what behaviours you'll allow or restrict in your recovery.**
2. **Do further research and reflection if you need.**
3. **Ask yourself, 'Is masturbation going to be helpful in my recovery?'**
4. **Talk over your answer with your accountability partner and anyone else supporting your recovery.**

CHAPTER FIVE: UNDERSTANDING YOUR ADDICTION CYCLE

Are you a science buff? If so, it's your lucky day! We're taking a short break from the emotional heavy lifting to delve into some objective knowledge and scientific research. This chapter focuses on the science of neurochemistry and brain plasticity. If you were more of an artsy-fartsy kid in school, like I was, don't worry—I won't take you too deep! This is a brief overview researched and written by an English nerd. I took the time to understand this content and included this chapter because it's important to get a grasp on how and why pornography affects a woman's brain; understanding this concept will provide you with the background needed to understand your personal addiction cycle, unique triggers and patterns which will make up the latter half of this chapter. It's important to understand these things, as they can become anchors for recovery. I know this from experience.

Before I realised that pornography actually affected my brain in a distinct way, my struggle felt out of control. The frequency of porn use and the intensity of my sexual desire felt unmanageable. I was constantly in the middle of a sex-tornado (not as fun as it sounds), my emotions were wild and I was frequently triggered seemingly out of the blue. Being able to identify how and why my brain was reacting to sexual stimuli, and knowing the four stages of the addiction cycle gave me the upper hand. It meant I could track and predict when I may be triggered to act out. It meant my crazed, out-of-control experience of addiction became calmer. I was less confused when I was able to relate my personal experiences to a predictable cycle and deconstruct what was going on for me in my body, mind and spirit. While I still struggled for some time, I was no longer at the mercy of porn as I once was. At least in my head, I had a clear understanding of why I was lapsing and how porn was tripping me up. It wasn't a mess anymore. It was simply a (very tough) challenge I was prepared to face and overcome. Attempting to overcome porn without a decent understanding of how it affects the brain is like eating soup with a fork.

So, get ready to engage your brain! Trust me, as we move along, there's going to be a lot of heart probing and emotional reflection. Enjoy this little break while it lasts and let's get practical!

Defining addiction

First off, let's define sex addiction (pornography is included in this definition).

According to Marnie Ferree, author of *No Stones: women redeemed from sexual addiction*[1] and founder of Bethesda Workshops: 'sexual addiction is the lack of control of some sexual behaviour or relationship. Perhaps the most helpful definition is a practical one: sexual or relational behaviour that has a negative effect on one's life.'[2] She also uses the four-component model of what comprises any addiction to identify sex and porn addicts:

1. Compulsivity
2. Continued use despite negative consequences

3. Preoccupation or obsession
4. Tolerance

The term sexual addiction is widely accepted and used within the world of recovery. It has helped many people understand their behaviours and seek effective support. However, the medical and psychiatric world at large are yet to welcome this term. At the time of publishing, sexual addiction is not currently listed in the Diagnostic and Statistical Manual of Mental Disorders (DSM). However, the World Health Organisation (WHO) did add Compulsive Sexual Behaviour Disorder (CSBD) to the 11th edition of the International Classification of Diseases (ICD-11) in 2018. CSBD is characterised by 'a persistent pattern of failure to control intense, repetitive sexual impulses or urges resulting in repetitive sexual behaviour'. According to its diagnostic description in the ICD-11; this can include both the act of sex and sexual fantasies[3]. While linguistically different, this definition appears to be a fitting and helpful classification for porn addicts seeking treatment from professionals.

An abundance of Christian 'addicts'

It is important to note the prevalence of Christian misdiagnosis before we move on. The term 'addiction' gets thrown around quite a lot in church. In our predominantly rule and shame-based purity culture, struggling with sex or pornography in any way is deemed one of the more serious sins. As such, the Church (certainly not every church, but in general) tends to lean towards using more serious language to describe the struggle; i.e. 'addiction'. In many of these cases, neither leaders or self-diagnosed addicts are qualified to make these claims.

Women are particularly susceptible to jumping the gun and identifying as addicts or being labelled as such simply because of miseducation. Women are often chastised for being vocal about their sex drives and curiosities, and are especially vulnerable to being diagnosed as 'masturbation addicts' if they participate in the behaviour regularly. Women are taught they shouldn't have sex drives or be visually stimulated—that's for men! So, when normal, healthy women find they are, or struggle semi-regularly, it's easy to wonder if something is wrong with them—are they addicted?

I'm not sharing this information to shame the Church or self-diagnosed addicts. God knows we have enough of that in Christian culture already! I simply want to be honest about the situation, and be respectful of the research that defines addiction. I want to clarify that not every woman who struggles with pornography (or masturbation) is an addict. Save those diagnoses for the professionals, and remain aware that there are certain guidelines required to be considered a legitimate porn addict. Habitual sin doesn't always necessarily equate to addiction, but it might.

Whether you fall into the 'addicted' category or not, you still need help. If you find yourself continually drawn to pornography and wanting to resist the urge because of your values but cannot—that's a problem. If you've viewed pornography only recently and find yourself wanting to go back in your head but your heart says otherwise, that's a problem. If you continue to use pornography, masturbation or other sexual behaviours to medicate feelings of pain more often than you'd like, you need support. You do not need to be at your lowest to seek support and recovery. Even casual porn use affects the brain and lays the foundation for a future of addiction. The following information is just as true for a casual porn user as it is the addict. The process which will be explained will simply be more deep-seated for the more frequent user. Catch issues before they become life-defining or addictive. Get help now.

With a definition of addiction in place, we can now delve deeper. How does addiction work? How does porn affect the brain? The following information has been sourced from Fight the New Drug[4].

Doctors and scientists used to believe in order for something to be addictive, it had to be a physical substance that was put into the body in some way. After researching the brain and how it reacts to addictive substances however, this common belief has changed dramatically. It is now understood it isn't as important what is put into the body, but rather how the brain reacts to it—specifically, how the reward pathway responds. For example, using cocaine or tobacco inserts new chemicals into the brain, but porn doesn't bring anything new. It just manipulates what already exists in your brain. The process under observation, however, is strikingly similar to that of hard drugs or cigarettes.

The reward pathway

Let's talk about that reward pathway. Everyone has one in their brain; its job is to motivate you to do things that protect and promote your survival—things like eating to stay alive or having sex to produce babies and continue the survival of the species. The way it rewards you for doing those things is by flooding your brain with dopamine and a cocktail of other 'pleasure' chemicals each time you do them. Your brain will even give you a micro dose of pleasure when you think about these things, just to remind you of how good you could feel if you take action on these thoughts!

The thing is though, your brain doesn't always lead you towards, or reward you for, the right things. For example, it produces higher levels of dopamine when you chow down on a pink iced donut than when you eat a trendy vegan salad. Weird, right? We'd all be so much healthier if we craved salads over donuts all the time! But our cave-woman design isn't so much interested in being slim, but rather eating lots of calories, especially the sugary, fatty kinds! All those years ago, our ancestors needed high calorie food to survive. They didn't come by them often, so their brains went into desire overload, sending the message: 'Eat, girl! Eat it all!'. Cave women didn't know when their next meal would come around, they had to take it when it arrived. That feeling is still so relatable today, isn't it? This is because the reward pathway hasn't changed, even though our food situation has. It's still in survival mode. If we listened to it every day, we'd end up with a lot of pink donuts in our bellies … and feeling pretty sick.

As with food, the same process is true of sex and pornography. The human brain is wired to crave sex—no surprises there, right? Now, you don't need sex to survive (although it may feel that way sometimes), but sex does ensure the survival of the gene pool. We are wired at a biological level to continue reproduction. But porn messes things up. Porn is akin to that high-calorie pink donut; it's sexual junk food. When a person is looking at porn, their brain is fooled into pumping out dopamine just as if they really were seeing a potential mate. Sure, filling your brain with feel-good chemicals might sound like a great idea at first, but just like with junk food, it's more dangerous than it seems.

Not only can you get yourself addicted to a screen, meaning you're missing out on genuine human connection and intimacy, but you can actually damage your brain and eventually rob yourself of pleasure. Porn overstimulates the reward centre in your brain. Viewing sex on screen is much more intense than real intercourse. The internet provides endless options for porn viewing, it gives you the ability to seamlessly switch between tabs and flash hundreds of different images across your vision in a single session. Online content has endless novelty, and some genres of porn are extreme and terrifying. All of this takes the warm-fuzzy sex chemicals to another level. Your brain becomes overstimulated, and the reward pathway is flooded with dopamine.

In an attempt to defend itself from the tsunami of chemicals, the brain releases one more: cyclic adenosine monophosphate response element binding protein, or CREB if you just got tongue tied. It acts like a set of emergency brakes on the crazy train that is your reward pathway. It does its best to slow the pleasure response right down by dulling the neurotransmitters that receive the pleasure signals. In doing this, the same amount of dopamine floods the brain but the person feels it less. It's like the difference between standing in a rain storm with or without an umbrella. The rain doesn't change, but the person feels the effects less.

Scientists have come to believe that CREB is partly why consumers have to keep increasing their porn intake to get aroused. That numbed-out state is called 'tolerance' and it's part of any kind of addiction. You might have experienced this yourself. Has your porn use escalated over time? For me, it started out as images, which turned to GIFs, which turned to explicit words, and eventually videos ... and the content became more and more intense as the years passed. It just didn't feel as good or exciting after a while. As porn consumers become desensitised from repeated overloads of dopamine, they often find they can't feel normal without a dopamine high. Even other things that used to make them happy, such as catching up with girlfriends, eating good food or physical activity aren't as enjoyable because of the dulling effect of CREB. Increased pornography use is the only thing that promises that old high.

Pornography has a stark impact on women's brains. I know we're all told that men are the visual ones, but when you put two brains on porn under the microscope, you'll find the foundations are the same. We all have a reward centre and porn hijacks it. Watching porn isn't simply a moral failing or lack of willpower; there are very real, and very powerful chemicals at play inside your brain. And not only do they come out to play once you're actually looking at porn, but they start to tingle and chat with each other before you even get there. Just as the chemicals in the reward pathway draw you towards pink donuts and other delicious things, they draw you towards porn. This begins before you're even conscious of it. From the slightest trigger, your brain starts to latch onto the idea of sex. Like a magnet, porn attracts your brain and draws it closer to acting out every moment. The reward centre is doing its job: drawing you towards and rewarding you for what it thinks is sex with a real mate.

Don't worry; there's hope!

Even though your brain is fizzing away with a cocktail of pleasure chemicals and doing its darn best to help you 'survive' by rewarding you for accessing pornography, you can change. You can experience freedom from pornography and outsmart your own brain!

The amazing thing about your brain is that it's plastic. No, there's not a scrunched-up plastic bag squashed into your skull, your brain is still made of pink squishy stuff, but *it is* mouldable. The brain can physically change. This means that continued use of pornography can alter your sexual tastes and perception of others, as well as develop into an addiction. But more importantly, brain plasticity means you can reverse this. You can heal. You can train your brain to live without pornography! It used to be believed that the brain was like a computer: once it was set or damaged, it couldn't be altered. This meant that addicts, trauma survivors or stroke patients had to deal with their lot in life—a broken brain. But research into neuroplasticity has developed a brand-new analogy: our brain is full of 'pathways'. Every time we participate in a behaviour, such as dancing, playing an instrument, using pornography (or actively choosing not to), our brains strengthen certain pathways[5]. Think of these neural pathways as bush tracks. At first, there will be obstacles as you traverse that path. It won't be the easiest route, but as you continue to walk that same path every day it will become easier. Your feet will create a clear pathway, and every time you wander down it, it becomes wider and easier to do so. If something bad happens on your bushwalk and you need to get home ASAP, you're going to take the easiest route, right? Why wade through an overgrown walkway when you could take the easy and familiar one?

Every time you use pornography, you walk the same neurological pathway and just like the bush track, that pathway becomes wider and easier to access every time you use it. It becomes the easiest route to pleasure, and the safest way 'home' after a negative experience throws you off your game. This is addiction. When you quit pornography though, and start to blaze new, healthy trails, that path will grow over. Eventually, it'll slip your mind and the days of compulsive, unwanted sexual behaviour will be behind you. You'll be hiking through trails of healthy connection and fulfilling hobbies!

In the next section, we'll be examining the addiction cycle in closer detail. Every completed cycle strengthens your 'porn pathway', so it's vital to understand the different stages and how to effectively interrupt them in order to place yourself on a different track.

The addiction cycle

Many women send emails and Facebook messages to me through The Grace Spot, but one in particular stands out. Harper, a twenty-eight-year-old woman shared her ten-year battle with pornography and masturbation with me. She told me how many times she had vowed to quit and how much she hated what she did. Her email was desperate, and the words I cannot forget were in capital letters at the end of her message:

'WHY CAN'T I JUST STOP?? WHAT THE HECK IS WRONG WITH ME??'

Have you ever asked the same question? How many times have you vowed you would never look at porn again, or refuse to look at a man lustfully … only to end up right back in the same place of addiction? I know how frustrating it is. No matter how much willpower and ferocity you throw into avoiding your acting out behaviour, it always seems to win. No matter what you try, you end up in the warm embrace of porn.

I know how distressing that feeling is, I experienced it for over ten years. But if you examine this continual draw to porn, and your past relapses, you'll actually see a picture of hope. Don't worry, I haven't gone crazy!

There's hope because there's a pattern. There always is. It's not a wild lack of willpower or moral failing that keeps you tangled up in porn. You're currently trapped in the addiction cycle, spinning around and around it like an old shirt in a washing machine. Not so pleasant, but when you know what's going on, you can get yourself out of there.

The addiction cycle was originally outlined by Dr Patrick Carnes[6], and is further explained in Marnie Ferree's book *No Stones*[7]. It is a predictable cycle that all addiction follows. There are five stages: trigger, fantasy, ritual, acting out and despair. The wounded self sits above the entire cycle. These stages identify the behavioural changes that occur during a lapse, as prompted by neurochemical responses to triggers.

With a grasp on how porn affects the brain on a neurological level, and the behaviours associated with the addiction cycle, you can piece together a predictable pattern. The benefit of identifying your personal patterns is that you can prepare yourself for what's to come. When you feel drawn to that familiar cycle, you can step out of it. You can interrupt the addiction cycle. You'll find an illustration of the addiction cycle on the following page.

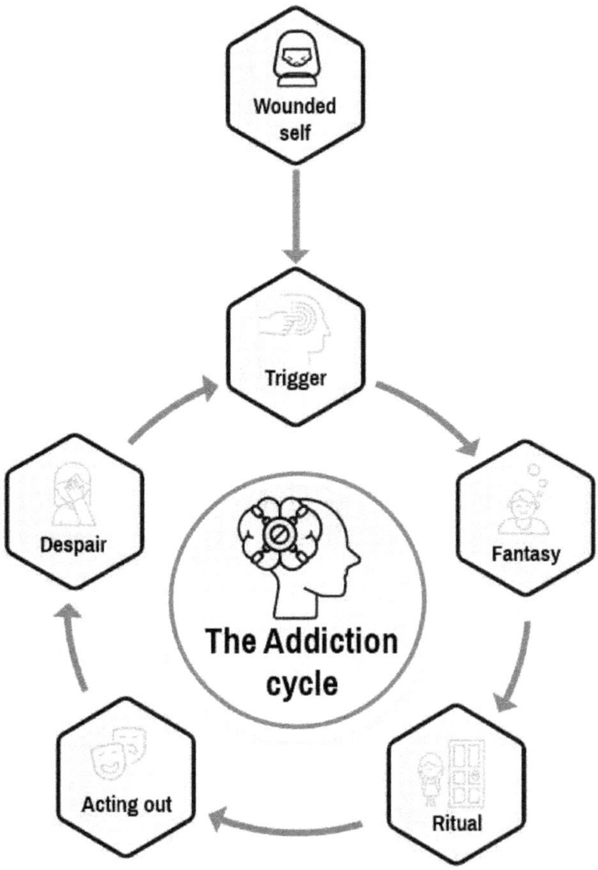

Let's look at each of these stages in closer detail:

The Wounded Self

The Wounded Self will be the focus of the following chapter, 'Reflection'. Understanding the wounds of the past and the pain you carry is so vital to recovery, it deserves its own chapter. As the graphic illustrates, it is the overarching cause and driving force behind the entire addiction cycle and where it all begins. We will be reflecting on this woundedness, and work on eliminating it later on, because once you cut off that first step, your chances of falling back into the cycle are greatly reduced!

For now, as you develop a fuller understanding of the cycle as a whole, just note that the Wounded Self refers to pain, discomfort or negative emotion. Feeling unsatisfied or outright distressed is the reason we seek out porn; we seek out the comfort that comes from the previously mentioned reward pathway. Dopamine, which is the warm-fuzzy-feel-good chemical, flows through your brain and body the moment you begin tantalising the idea of sex—on screen or in real life. That sure as hell feels better than sitting around feeling cold, low and overwhelmed, doesn't it? It makes sense. In our discomfort or pain, we seek the comfort of escape. In our loneliness, porn appears to offer easy intimacy.

Once you have read through chapter six it may be helpful to return to this graphic and note the ways you specifically experience woundedness, shame or pain. For example, you may write 'feeling rejected', 'anger at my parents lack of kindness', 'dwelling on my singleness', or 'feeling sad' atop your personal addiction cycle.

Triggers

Triggers bring the addiction cycle to life. There are two types: pleasure triggers and pain triggers. Both of these cause a neurological reaction, and can throw you right into the addiction cycle.

Pleasure triggers may be more obvious—these are anything that prompt sexual fantasy. Glaring examples include sexually provocative advertisement, billboards, sex scenes in movies, music videos, books, lingerie ads and straight up porn which seems to pop up and be more accessible than oxygen these days! Shopping centres are a minefield of pleasure triggers for a woman struggling with pornography.

Stepping down from the obvious sexually explicit triggers women face in the twenty first century, there are more individual pleasure triggers women will come across during their recovery. These are things which have a positive sexual association to you, such as the smell of a certain cologne or lotion, a song, outfit, or a person with sexual memories attached to them. They are things which remind you of previous experiences of intimacy. These may go completely unseen by any other woman, but to you, they are loaded with meaning and desire. Inanimate objects can become pleasure triggers as well, things like laptops, particular settings (e.g. your study or bedroom) or lotions and sex toys used in the acting out process. Over time, those trusty brain chemicals mentioned earlier begin to associate these objects with a hit of dopamine and pleasure, so simply sighting or thinking about them causes a neurochemical reaction. And the more you dwell, the more intense it gets, and suddenly what began as a trickle has turned into a raging river of desire, and you're being carried with it.

All these things are like magnets for dopamine. As discussed earlier, the reward pathway is designed to draw humans towards survival activities such as sex. As soon as something even remotely sexual comes into sight, those rewarding pleasure chemicals begin moving through your brain and can be incredibly difficult to ignore.

Pain triggers are far more complex to deconstruct, but just as important to understand. Doing so will give you the gift of preparedness so you can have the best defences possible.

Woundedness, discomfort and pain overarch and fuel the cycle; each woman has unique pain and different levels of hurt. These wounds often come from ruptured intimacy, trauma, abuse, neglect or childhood pain. These can manifest in fear, anger, depression, paranoia, mistrust or broken relationships.

A pain trigger is anything that makes us acutely aware of these painful memories and emotions. Anything that tears open that old wound, making it bleed. In this moment, our pain is enhanced and brought to our attention, and it demands to be anaesthetised. It hurts, it's overwhelming, and escaping into fantasy seems to be the best and quickest option to avoiding this fresh pain.

Triggers with negative associations cut deeper than pleasure triggers. These are things that remind you of a painful memory or emotion. They can be seen, heard, felt, smelled, tasted, remembered or brought up by another person's comment or actions. For example, seeing a photo on Instagram of a social gathering you weren't invited to can bring up feelings of rejection. Rejection on its own can hurt, but often it goes much deeper. That feeling of rejection could be attached to a painful or traumatic event in your life, such as a break up or parent leaving. A woman who has lost her mother to cancer or another illness may find herself triggered by a movie that touches on familiar medical memories. This may trigger feelings of abandonment and grief. These emotions can spiral out of control. General stress, sickness or pain are also prominent negative triggers. Two helpful acronyms for identifying general triggers are HALT (hungry, angry, lonely, tired) and BLASTS (bored, lonely, angry, stressed, tired, shamed). These feelings suck, and your brain remembers how to make you feel good again: that familiar cycle of seeking out and using pornography.

If you've been struggling with porn for long enough and have done some kind of reflection, you may have a good idea of what some of your triggers are. If you don't, you can often discern a trigger by gauging if your emotional reaction to a particular event seems out of proportion or has spiralled far too rapidly. If you've experienced a lapse, it helps to reflect back on the events leading up to it, the hours, day and even week prior. What got your emotions flaring? What stressors were you experiencing? What or who did you want to get away from? What was different this week? Was anything particularly emotional on your mind? This is a great task to share with an accountability partner, as they may have insight from doing day to day life with you, too.

Can you see now that what you see, smell, experience and remember are all connected? It's not as random as you once thought when you sit down and pay attention. When you identify your personal triggers, you can put precautions and boundaries in place to avoid succumbing to their lure. You need to do the same with the rest of the cycle, too. After a trigger comes fantasy, ritual, acting out and despair.

Fantasy

Fantasy is also referred to as 'preoccupation'. This is the first stage of the cycle after being triggered. It is a trance-like state where you begin to think sexual thoughts and dwell on them. You tantalise yourself with the idea of acting out, and the way it will make you feel. This stage is the gateway to a full-on lapse, as you start to dip your mental toes in the water and think 'Maybe I could …', 'Last time felt so good …', 'Nobody is home …'. You are entering fantasy-land, and your thoughts are engrossed with sex.

Already, your brain is beginning to react to the sexual thoughts. Dopamine is shaking off its slumber and starting to buzz. At just stage one of the cycle you are already experiencing a neurochemical 'high'. The cycle will only speed up and intensify from here on.

Rituals

There's nothing religious or spiritual about this phase. Rituals simply refer to any repeated behaviours that lead up to your sexual acting out. These are different for every single person, and includes anything that transitions you from fantasy to acting out. For example, you may shut the door, close the blinds and turn 'incognito' mode on your laptop before looking at porn. Another ritual may involve fetching a certain lotion or sex toy. Some are longer, and involve other people. For example, putting a sexy pair of underwear on and shaving your legs before meeting a tinder date may be part of a longer ritual involving having sex with another person. It is vital to identify your personal rituals so you can grow in self-awareness and cut them off before they begin.

Once you begin your ritual, it is almost certain you will act out. You've been thrown head-first into the addiction cycle and it's near-impossible to escape, until you are dumped out the other end, in despair and shame.

What are your normal rituals? For me, I closed the door, curtains and went on incognito mode. I turned on the laptop or phone and typed in the words I knew would lead me down a path to pleasure.

Acting out

This is the part of addiction you're probably most familiar with. It may feel like this is where it starts, but as you can see, there are at least two phases before this that have been leading up to it. This is almost the finale! Every woman has a different way of acting out. It may involve masturbation, pornography, cybersex or acting out with another person in reality. It may involve many more things. In your inventory, you identified the ways in which you act out.

Despair

This one's familiar right? After the euphoria of acting out and escaping for a little while, you come crashing down. It's your porn (or masturbation or sex) hangover. At the end of the cycle, you feel chewed up, spat out and completely helpless and hopeless against this addiction. Your worst fears about yourself are confirmed: 'I am a bad, unworthy person. I am disgusting. I won't ever get free.' This is a point of extreme and poignant shame. This shame adds to your existing woundedness, and feeds right back into the cycle over and over again. The despair you feel after acting out demands to be anaesthetised, and you find yourself triggered by your own porn use, into acting out the entire addiction cycle again. Beginning and end merge into one, and you feel trapped in a seemingly everlasting cycle of pain, shame, medication and despair. And every time you cycle through, the pathways in your brain become stronger and more familiar. Your pattern of behaviour is creating a super highway.

Interrupt the cycle

In order to overcome pornography addiction, you must learn to interrupt the addiction cycle. This is achieved by knowing your wounded self, identifying your unique triggers, and understanding the ways the four stages of the cycle manifest in your life and feed into one another. Awareness is the key to interrupting the addiction cycle. The best way to interrupt the cycle is to call in outside help. Hello, accountability partner! When your brain is dying to hit auto pilot, and you feel on the verge of losing control, call your accountability partner(s) and let them know you need support. The simple act of stopping, acknowledging what's going on and physically calling for help can be enough to interrupt the cycle. It takes your mind away from preoccupation and distracts you from beginning rituals which will inevitably lead to acting out and despair. It's wise to invite your accountability partner to check in on you a few hours later, too. This can act as a safeguard and motivation to abstain from porn. If temptation lingers after your initial accountability check in, keep interrupting the cycle, no matter how many times it tries to start up again. Be intentional about distracting yourself and stepping out of that trap. Start by acknowledging whatever stage you are in—are you feeling wounded or triggered? Are you actively fantasising, ritualizing or acting out? Once you identify this, you can change the ending. Choose something better. Some examples women have shared with me include:

- Go for a run
- Head to the gym and lift weights
- Visit a friend or invite them over
- Call your parents (nothing fizzles desire like talking to family!)
- Bake a cake
- Clean the house
- Pray, read the Bible or listen to worship music
- Get creative: paint, draw, and other arts and craft
- Sit outside

- Plan an event
- Meal prep for the week
- Go to the local shopping centre or grocery store
- Go for a long drive
- Laughing meditation
- Blast some fun music and sing or dance along
- Weed and water your garden
- Play with a pet

Remember, you can interrupt the addiction cycle at any stage. Statistically, once ritualising begins it is extremely unlikely the individual will stop before acting out and injecting the cycle with more despair and shame, but it's not impossible! Even if you've already burned through fantasy, rituals, and have started to watch porn or act out in any way, you can stop. You can stop in the middle of a porn session, and you'll be doing good by yourself. Often, it can feel too late to stop. Women think 'Well I'm already here now, I've already sinned or been bad, I may as well finish' or they know the despair that comes when it all ends, and figure they may as well experience some short pleasure before it hits. The reality is, every time you interrupt the cycle before it naturally comes to completion (and starts again), you are changing your brain. You are getting stronger, and creating new neural pathways which remind you that you can say no to porn. You're also avoiding the despair and shame that comes after acting out. It's never too late to interrupt the cycle, but it sure as hell is easier if you catch it early on.

Menstrual cycle

We've talked about a lot of cycles in this chapter. I hope your head isn't spinning! But there's another very important, uniquely feminine cycle that we should discuss here: the menstrual cycle. The best thing about periods (is there a best thing?), is that they are another predictable cycle you can utilise in your recovery (that is, if your period is generally punctual).

You may have noticed that about two weeks before your period is due, you're much more sexually aware and tempted. I know I experience this! When I was single and struggling to overcome masturbation and porn, I could manage to go three or so weeks without my vice, but my menstrual hormones would come rushing in and my body was out of control. I was like the incredible horny hulk. It was physically unbearable. I'd have sex dreams and even become aroused listening to a male radio presenter's voice.

How does it work?

I'm not sure what your sex education was like in school, but mine was pretty feeble (all I remember is feeling mortified having to discuss safe sex with my crush sitting nearby). I actually learned so much more about my own reproductive system through my studies in agriculture!

Our class spent an entire term learning about the reproductive system of cows. One particular female substitute teacher took the syllabus to a whole new level by relating our animal studies to our own bodies. It turns out, humans don't go into 'heat' like our four-legged friends. We are interested in sex for recreation and can reproduce all year around. However, a woman's time of fertility comes around once a month, during ovulation. This is an approximately six-day window where she can get pregnant. This is called the 'fertile window', but I also like to call it the 'temptation window'. If you've ever worked on a farm, you'll know that when animals are in 'heat' (their fertile time) they go a little sex-crazy and start participating in weird behaviours. Not that I'm calling you a cow, but there are some similarities! Like in the animal kingdom, our biological purpose is to reproduce. Our wonderfully made bodies know this, and hit us with a boost of testosterone and other hormones (read: a big dose of sex drive) once a month.

It's just our bodies helpful little way of making sure we get pregnant when we can. Pretty cool, huh? But not when you're struggling with addiction!

You may have also noticed that about a week before menstruation, you experience moodiness, pain, fatigue and a host of other unpleasant symptoms which act as warning bells for your body: 'Your period is coming! Prepare!'. If you remember the addiction cycle, you'll know it doesn't exist without woundedness or discomfort. These physical and emotional pre-menstrual symptoms can act as triggers which push us into the old cycle of acting out. You feel like crap; you want to escape. Simple. This is another time of the month you should be conscious of, and preparing for with self-care, rest and accountability.

Our menstrual cycle is a unique tool we can tap into as women. It provides yet another predictable and trackable cycle you can use to stay on your guard against temptation and weakness. If you're interested in finding out more about the menstrual cycle and fertility, head to any pregnancy or conception website—they have lots of graphics and calendars to help you understand your body. The simplest thing to remember though, is that fertile equals sex drive.

With this information in hand, it's time to track your period! There are many ways to track your period and fertility. The easiest option is to simply download a period tracking app on your phone, or use your calendar to note the phases of your cycle. The benefit of apps is you can track symptoms, events and details in one private place, and they often alert you to your fertile (temptation) window by notification. But a good old paper calendar will also do the trick. You'll find by doing this over a few months, you'll not only save quite a few pairs of underwear from getting ruined, but also grow a helpful awareness of the workings of your body, and when you're more likely to succumb to temptation.

Conclusion

There are cycles all around us as women, and we can use them to our advantage. Learning about and understanding how your hormones impact daily life, and the specific stages of the addiction cycle, gives you an upper hand in recovery. This knowledge turns chaos into order. When you can predict what's coming you have the power to utilise your understanding and recovery tools to put boundaries in place and seek help before you relapse. Preparedness is power.

Action Steps:

1. **Download, print out or draw your own addiction cycle. Customise it with your personal triggers, fantasies, rituals, acting out behaviours and what despair looks like in you. You can download the addiction cycle from The Grace Spot, under the heading 'Get Help' followed by 'Download Worksheets' which you'll find under 'Read my Book' or at thegracespot.com/Restored-worksheets.**

2. **On the same image, use a different coloured pen to list when and how you can interrupt the cycle. This is your plan of action in times of temptation. What activities can you do to break the cycle of addiction?**
3. **If you menstruate, download a period tracking app or use a calendar to track your cycle.**

CHAPTER SIX: REFLECTION

So far, if you've been following this guide, you've shared your sexual struggle with a trusted friend or mentor, you've done an inventory of your sexual acting out and habits, you've considered where you might sit on the masturbation debate and have recently examined your personal addiction cycle. You've identified what makes you tick, what your rituals are and how you act out. There's been a lot of talk about sex, hasn't there? Which may seem pretty obvious since that's what your struggle is all about ... right?

Well, actually that's not *quite* right. While you definitely do struggle with pornography and sexual behaviours, these aren't the primary issue you need to deal with. They're simply a symptom of something deeper that's going on in your life.

Does reading this stir anything in you?

Are you aware, even in a foggy or hidden sense that the real issue has something to do with your heart and your history?

Have you ever considered looking beyond the porn use, and asking yourself *why* you compulsively use it?

Whether you have had any inkling that there's something else going on, whether you definitely know it but have been in denial, or the raging war against pornography in your life has been too distracting to even consider anything but the actual thing that tempts you, this is your invitation to let the walls down and compassionately reflect on your heart. This is a call to let your eyes see beyond the surface behaviours, beyond the addiction, no matter how painful it is. This is your chance to examine the state of your heart, without judgement, danger or shame.

Does this idea make you nervous? Do you want to skip this section and just find a filter that will keep porn out of your life? Do you believe me when I say there's more to it than simply your compulsive porn use? If you're a sceptic right now, that probably means this chapter was written for you. You picked up this book for a reason, you owe it to yourself to read every chapter and try every exercise. What do you have to lose? Aside from a wounded heart and a porn addiction?

Wherever you're at in the journey, and no matter how broken or whole your heart may feel right now, this isn't going to be easy. Healing never is. Each reader will have a different experience, but it may feel like getting cut open all over again. It may feel sharp and painful at times. The memories may revive fresh feelings of shame, guilt, fear, anger or any mix of emotions imaginable. As that wound begins to stitch itself together again, it will scab over. It will itch, it will bother, it may break open again if it needs. You will be aware of it—which may be difficult if you've spent most of your life tucking it away under a bandaid and ignoring it. When we have wounds, they hurt when they happen, and they hurt as they heal. There's no use putting it off, let's get into it. Let's compassionately and gently examine the root cause of your addiction to pornography, and get started on a truly healing trajectory.

It's not just a porn problem; it's an intimacy disorder

Women who struggle with porn don't just have a 'sex issue'. They have an intimacy disorder.

Georgia says: *When my [online erotica] readers didn't satisfy my desire to be validated, I found my way to pornographic chat rooms where I would speak with men, lie about my age and engage in cybersex with them over webcam, doing whatever they commanded of me and my body. I still remember the things I did for the sake of their approval. I just wanted to be wanted. I wanted someone to tell me that I was desirable, and these men did that for me. These readers of the erotic fiction I wrote did it. It was all I thought about.*

Similarly, Summer says: *I was desperate to feel desired. I wanted to be noticed, pursued and wanted. I craved physical touch like nothing else. In my mind, sex equalled love so I sought out a fantasy world in porn. I watched people having sex and let myself imagine I was the woman in the video. I was the centre of attention, the men wanted me more than anything. They wanted to be with me, touch me. It wasn't really about the sex; it was about the feeling of being desired. It was about finding some kind of worth.*

Nia says: *When I used porn and fantasied, I imagined I was the women in the videos who made the guys go crazy, so crazy they abused her. I fantasised that someone wanted me enough to pursue me, that just looking at my body would make them putty in my hands. I dreamed of non-sexual touch, companionship, unconditional love, someone to protect me. I was so starved of intimacy, and I was seeking it in all the wrong places.*

More than anything else these women wanted to be validated, desired and pursued. They craved acceptance, approval, touch and love. They weren't simply seeking an orgasm, there was something more important at stake. Summer said it herself, it wasn't really about the sex at all. It was about manufacturing the feeling of intimacy. All the words they used to describe their innermost needs could easily be swapped out with that one word: intimacy.

But why do these women so desperately seek it? And why do they feel the need to use pornography and sex as a means to achieve it, rather than finding a friend or partner to share intimacy with? Well, it's because they missed out somewhere along the line. At some point in their past life or ongoing experience, the comfort of safe relationship either was, or felt, unavailable. In lieu of human connection, these women seek out a virtual fantasy realm where intimacy is available to all through sex. The problem is though, when you view porn, you're not looking at intimacy, you're looking for it.

The loss of intimacy

Experiencing an absence of intimacy can be gargantuan in impact. Humans were created for connection; from the moment you were conceived, your life depended on the intimacy of being inside your mother's womb. From first breath, your survival counted on that same connection and safekeeping. Multiple studies have shown repeated human interaction like touching, cuddling, talking and eye contact makes newborn babies release hormones which help their brain to grow. This intentional connection also creates the foundation for their emotional wellbeing. They feel safe enough to play, explore and face setbacks later in life. Babies and children who experience adequate levels of parent-child intimacy are often healthier, more emotionally intelligent and more resilient adults[1]. These adults function best in life when they share connection with a wide range of people, too. Friends and community were never intended to be harmful, but to be a source of joy, and spouses were made to become 'one' and share intimacy in a sacred and safe way.

It's in your blood to share intimacy with other humans, in both sexual and non-sexual ways. Intimacy is emotional oxygen. Without a healthy expression of connection, we begin to suffocate.

This is why when this need is left unmet or distorted for any number of reasons at any stage of life, it is human instinct to go out and seek it at all costs. As a starved person is prone to binging on food when it does become available, so too will the intimacy starved girl or woman live in overdrive. She will crave closeness, affirmation, validation, physical touch and experience an overwhelming need to be desired. It will be the subject of many-a-fantasy, it will consume her thoughts and become the primary lens through which she views the world and makes decisions.

Females with intimacy disorders may seek to fill that gaping hole with a number of compulsive behaviours. Drinking, taking drugs, excessive spending, shoplifting or overeating are common escapes from the pain of loss. They are especially vulnerable to falling into addictive and unhealthy sexual behaviours, though. Women with distorted experiences of intimacy often find themselves trapped in a cycle of pornography, masturbation, fantasy, overwhelming romantic obsessions or compulsive sex. Not only is the dopamine hit a welcome escape from the emotional pain of rejection, but sex sells itself as the 'safest' way to experience quick intimacy. There's no vulnerability required, yet you are promised satisfaction. It promises to deliver on what you missed out on.

But the world has lied to us about sex. It says that sex equals intimacy, love, validation and status.

Sex isn't intimacy. Intimacy is vulnerability, safety, being completely known and loved and being protected. It is trust and honesty between families, friends or lovers. Sex can certainly be an expression of this, but in and of itself, the act does not necessarily equate to intimacy. In fact, it can be the opposite. Sex with another person or on screen can rob you of your sense of worth and ability to connect.

Many of us will know this deeply. The thrill and promise of intimacy and affection throw us into the arms of pornography, lovers, or our own fantasies. Our intense desire to be wanted wraps us up and takes us into a fantasy realm—but upon re-entry into reality we realise it was all a lie. We are left unsatisfied, ashamed and feeling further away from genuine connection than ever. This only compounds our desire for intimacy. Again, it is ripped from our hands, so we run after it again to comfort the pain of its loss and desperately try to hold onto it. It is a dreadful cycle.

But there *is* a way out of this cycle! Genuine intimacy can be restored to your life and you can be freed from shame. The following chapters are full of practical tips on how to deal with an intimacy disorder, but there's more you need to understand, first. Before jumping ahead to the solution, allow yourself to look deeper and continue to reflect on the 'why' behind your struggle with porn. Absent or ruptured intimacy is the glue that holds your addictive cycle together and keeps it running. In order to heal you must understand what people or events influenced your experience of intimacy and what you have come to believe about yourself because of these. Once you are aware of these influences, you can begin to push back on them. That's where we're heading next.

The Tree

The best way to understand the underlying issues of a woman struggling with pornography is to picture an apple tree. This illustration is important as it goes beyond simply identifying behaviours, to reveal beneath the surface. The three components to the tree are the fruit, roots and soil.

1. **The Fruit** is the behaviour exhibited.

These are the most obvious elements to the tree, and as such, many women get stuck up here. It is common for women to focus only on the behaviours, but in doing so they forget the rest of the problem. Just like a real plant, in order for fruit to grow the plant must have roots, soil and nourishment.

2. **The Roots** are your core beliefs.

These are your beliefs about yourself, the world and those around you. These are beneath the surface and harder to see, but can be just as toxic as the fruit above. Without strong roots, the fruit of addiction couldn't grow.

3. **The Soil** is your environment.

Whatever is in your environment will nourish the roots (your core beliefs). The soil represents your upbringing and life experiences. In the case of porn addiction and ruptured intimacy, the soil is your painful experiences.

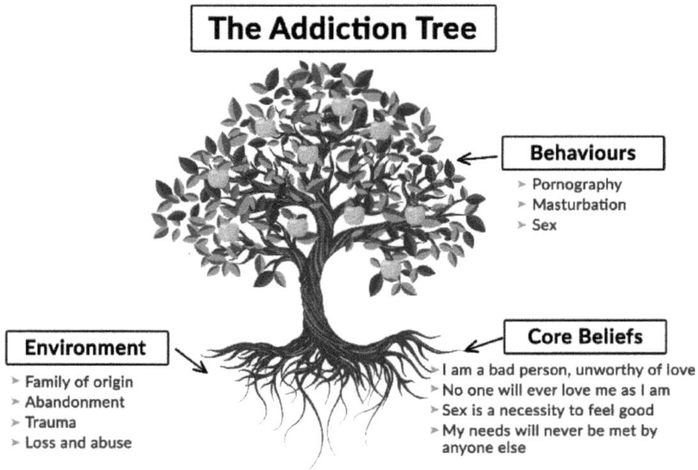

The tree analogy shows that you may be able to pluck the fruit off for a season but if those pesky roots are still intact—or remain in traumatic soil—the fruit will grow again next season. If you want to rid yourself of the fruit of porn addiction for good, you must uproot the tree and replace it with healing soil and fresh roots. It must be nurtured. And just like in horticulture, it may take some grit, dirt and sweat (and tears) to pull those roots up! But you've got this. A little hard work never scared you, did it?

Reflecting on the 'soil'. What's in your environment?

We started at the very top, examining your specific troublesome behaviours. Bear with me for a moment, while we go underground. We're going beneath the surface to identify your environment. What soil does your tree grow in? What was it like growing up, before those roots grew strong and solid? What remains in that hidden environment that continues to pump your tree with what it needs to produce addictive fruit? In human

terms, this is about examining and reflecting on the pain you may have experienced, both growing up and in the present. The pain of damaged intimacy. No matter if you were told 'it's normal', 'your fault' or 'in your head', it is important to name the beast and know you didn't deserve the hurt that happened to you. Healing toxic soil is the first step in restoring that tree to something with beautiful, healthy fruit.

Not everyone has obvious pain. The discomforts and complications of your life may be subtle, your experience of alienation unseen by others. This doesn't make your struggle any less valid, or any less powerful in directing you towards some form of medication, i.e. pornography. You don't need to have experienced traumatic pain in your life to find yourself experiencing an intimacy disorder and compulsive pornography use. In fact, you may struggle to identify any pain at all besides the trauma of pornography itself, or perhaps vicarious pain. Sensitive women (such as myself) are susceptible to feeling the effects of these deeply. Your pain is still valid. We'll be moving on to examine four areas of woundedness that most women struggling with intimacy and porn share. Each woman will identify with different aspects of these, and to varying degrees. Remember, just because someone else might feel pain differently to you doesn't mean your own experience is invalid. Another's pain doesn't cancel out yours, even if it feels insignificant in comparison.

The following four categories of emotional injury can predispose women to addictive behaviours. Examine them and reflect on how your own experience compares. These are deep and complex matters, which I am only able to give a brief overview of in this book. If you identify strongly with any or many of these, please discuss it with a professional therapist, and pursue further information on the topic. Dr Patrick Carnes[2] and Marnie Ferree[3] discuss them in detail in their books. The purpose of this list isn't to diagnose and do deep trauma work, it is simply to help you identify what may be going on for you under the porn addiction. I want to help you identify what you need further support in. I am no messiah, I cannot heal you all or save you from your intimacy issues, but I hope to shed light on them and point you to further support.

Family of Origin

It is said that pain travels through families, until someone is willing to feel it. This is why we are beginning our reflection with examining your family of origin.

Family woundedness is significant and common and can leave women with twisted core beliefs regarding her worth and ability to function within a community. Our parents and other family members have a mighty influence over our lives as vulnerable children growing up, and still as grown adults. They are our first experience of love, intimacy and safety. Unfortunately, they can also be our first experience of exploitation, pain and disappointment. It's likely that any woman looking back on her upbringing will have issues and baggage. That's part of life, no parent is all good or all bad, and most will make mistakes that have to be worked through to some degree by the adult child. There are, however, healthier and less healthy families. This is not about blame, but identifying where you've been hurt, and what work needs to be done there. That is not a nasty thing to do, but an honourable task; to seek truth and healing no matter what your family may say.

Consider the following questions, remembering to take them slowly and as you feel ready, and to reach out for support if the pain is too deep.

- What happy memories do you have of your family? What makes them special?
- How is your relationship with your family today?
- Are you aware of how your family impacts your current struggles?
- How did experiences in your childhood negatively impact you?
- Did you have boundaries in your family? Were they too loose or too rigid (or both)?
- Do you feel anger or resentment towards any family members? Why?
- Were your feelings dismissed growing up?
- Were you punished for expressing emotions?
- Did you walk on eggshells at home?
- Was either caregiver an addict?
- Did you feel loved growing up?
- Did you take on the role of peacekeeper? Joker? Surrogate spouse or rebel?
- Did you miss out on a childhood?
- Did your family give you distorted views of sex?

Trauma

Trauma is anything that overwhelms your brains ability to cope. When you think of trauma, something obvious and clear may pop up in your mind. You may think of overt abuse, a physical attack, a deeply horrific event or catastrophe. Maybe you think of a warzone. All these are certainly traumatic, and they may be your experience. But if you're not identifying with this, or you have a pain in your life that you dismiss because 'it shouldn't be such a big deal', remember trauma isn't always obvious. Trauma isn't always a 'big' event. Trauma can start off 'small' and be amplified by other events or experiences. Porn itself can act as the traumatising agent, especially when a person is exposed to it in childhood without explanation or support. This is an ever-increasing reality as pornography becomes more accessible and acceptable within society. Traditionally, professionals considered conventional childhood trauma necessary for a sexual addiction diagnosis. However, the accessibility and content of modern pornography is now more than capable of doing the traumatising itself and getting vulnerable people hooked.

Never disregard trauma because it doesn't seem 'big' or 'bad' enough. If your brain couldn't cope with what happened, if it has an ongoing impact on you and keeps you stuck in that memory or fear, it's trauma and it's okay to call it that. Your trauma is not vetoed by a war vet's bomb attack.

Trauma is a psychological injury. It requires treatment just as a broken arm would. Trauma sets your soil up for dysfunction.

Abandonment

Abandonment can be another form of trauma, but it deserves its own space as it is often overlooked. This is because it is an absence—of love, presence, nurturing or touch. If this environment is the only thing a woman has known, it can be difficult to identify what they haven't received. It is much easier to identify overt abuse or actions that cause direct physical harm.

It is important to note the effects of abandonment though. Deprivation is what leads to attachment issues, which can easily turn into obsession, compulsion and eventually addiction. Women who feel abandoned will seek touch, affirmation and intimacy. Often it is sought in harmful places, as the nature of their abandonment meant they were never taught safe and real connection.

Abandonment trauma, while often not recognised, can occur emotionally, sexually, physically and spiritually. It can be the effect of death, wilful or unknown neglect, divorce, lack of nurturing or outright abandonment.

To classify as abandonment, it doesn't have to be deliberate and cruel either. For example, in Russell Brand's book *Recovery* he identifies with feelings of abandonment and loss, resulting in resentment towards his mother who became ill with cancer[4]. Clearly, she did not do this out of spite, but young Russell legitimately and genuinely felt a sense of abandonment and resentment towards her, which he carried into his adult life and addictions. I experienced a similar sense of feeling deserted by my father. He was physically present and never caused me intentional harm but was unable to emotionally connect with me, and remains so. To me, this felt like abandonment.

Let this remind you that even if you weren't willingly or cruelly abandoned by your caregivers or anyone else, you may still feel that way—and that is valid. You may feel abandoned just as intensely as a literal orphan, even though your family loves you dearly in their own way. The trouble with this unintentional abandonment is the guilt that follows. It may be internal or it may come directly from family or friends, those who say 'Your life was normal, you weren't abused, you don't have it so bad! Get over it!'. Girl, you do not need to feel guilty. I don't care if your parents are the shiniest, most popular, power-pastor couple in the universe—if you feel abandoned in any sense of the word, you need to get support for that. This is impacting your life. This hurt. Whether it was a sick, injured or incapable parent who let you down, a deliberate abandonment, addicted parent, a break-up, loss by death, loss of friendship or a pet running away from home—your pain is valid, and acknowledging this will pave the way to healing.

- Describe how you feel abandoned
- Have you ever felt guilty for this feeling?
- In an ideal world, what would the relationship between you and whoever let you down look like?

Loss

Loss shares many characteristics with abandonment and can be tied up with family of origin issues and trauma. You may feel loss from a death, divorce, broken relationship, loss of a pet or friend, moving homes or estrangement from a lover or family member. You may also feel significant loss over a sentimental item, career or lost dream. Perhaps it is the loss of your health, youth or abilities. It may be a person or physical item you have lost, or it may be something more intangible, too. As a child or an adult, you may have lost, or felt robbed of, your security, dignity, safety, choice or trust. All these things impact us in different and significant ways, and are generally associated with some form of relationship. When we experience loss, when something is taken away or willingly leaves, we feel weak, vulnerable and powerless. Feelings of fear, shame and rejection thrive. You do what you can to avoid feeling this way again—this often means women go into hiding. In isolation, there's no risk of being hurt again. When you disconnect from reality, there's less to lose. This emotional environment leads women straight into the arms of pornography.

- What have you lost?
- What was taken from you as a child or adult?

Abuse

Abuse can occur physically, emotionally, sexually and spiritually. All four categories are as serious and impactful as each other and always involve another person or persons. Abuse is a mighty and dangerous experience, scarring women for life and distorting their view of intimacy. Abuse takes intimacy and tortures it, forever tarnishing genuine human connection and making it a thing of fear and pain. White Ribbon Australia[5] defines four common categories of abuse as follows:

Physical abuse happens when a person uses physical force against another. Physical abuse can start slowly and inconspicuously, for example with throwing an object or a slap, and get more intense or worse over time.

Emotional abuse does not leave physical scars but has a huge impact on a person's mental health. It includes name calling, exaggerated blame, humiliation, yelling, controlling behaviours (including what the person wears, who they associate with and how much money they can access), guilting them into behaviours and intimidation. Someone experiencing emotional abuse can feel anxious, depressed and even suicidal. Perpetrators of emotional abuse use it to take away a person's independence, confidence and self-esteem. This helps the perpetrator maintain power and control in the relationship. Physically abusive relationships often include aspects of emotional abuse.

Sexual abuse is any form of forced or unwanted sexual activity. The perpetrator of sexual abuse may use physical force, make threats or take advantage of a person unable to give consent. This also includes image-based abuse, where intimate digital content is shared without consent.

Spiritual abuse is the denial or use of spiritual or religious beliefs and practices to control and dominate a person. Spiritual abuse can impact on a someone's self-esteem and confidence, make them feel guilty, damage their spiritual experiences, and isolate them.

In any abuse situation, in order to sustain the power dynamic, the abuser will not only dominate the person in question but manipulate them into believing they are the cause of the abuse. They will transfer responsibility and guilt onto the person being abused, in order to sustain the pattern of abuse and prevent intervention or calling for help.

If you have experienced any abuse, at any time in your life, it is important to find your voice now, and speak out about it. It is important to acknowledge you were abused and wronged, and it was never your fault. The first step to healing is identifying what happened to you and removing your feelings of personal responsibility. Then, you must consult a professional counsellor or therapist to work through the trauma of these events. If you are currently in danger, you must do what you can to remove yourself from that environment, too.

The pain in our heart and histories is the issue. Broken relationships are at the core of your struggle. Using porn and other compulsive behaviours (eating, shopping, spending—ring a bell for you?) is simply surviving. You are anaesthetising your pain and coping how you know best. You are seeking a painkiller. Who wouldn't want to? Pain and isolation suck. But, dear woman, there is another way. There is a way to truly heal those wounds so they no longer scream at you, so they no longer fight to be anaesthetised. You don't need to cover it up anymore … you can be free. You need to excavate these old wounds, examine them with gentle care and replace the gaping holes they leave with intimacy, restored relationships, and lifegiving things. That will be the topic of the rest of this guide, but before then, let's have a look at the core beliefs which arise from our traumas and losses.

What are the roots of your addiction?

As the tree diagram demonstrated, your behaviours are the fruit that is most clearly seen. It comes back every season as long as the tree stands as it is and remains in the same state of care.

The soil is the environment the tree was planted in, and grows from. These are your family wounds, trauma, abuses, losses and experiences of pain and damaged relationships.

The final piece of the puzzle are the roots. These roots suck up nutrients and life from the soil, and take whatever is in that environment up to the surface. They are the vehicle through which the wounded environment impacts everyday life and behaviours. The roots are your core beliefs. These are ways in which you understand, explain and process the pain of your environment (either past or present). They are statements which you believe of yourself, your world and those around you.

As with all living plants, in the beginning the tree is small and weak. Its roots are thin and sporadic, shooting little green pops of colour as it grows. Our beliefs may start out as stray thoughts or a small voice in our mind, but as time goes on and the environment doesn't change, or even gets worse, those roots will grow. They will become thick and strong with conviction. They will become grounded, to a point where you simply cannot just dig them up and dispose of them. You have to overturn the entire system you've developed for understanding your world and start anew.

Let's look at what those roots are. Of course, as I always say, we are all unique in our addictions, but there are four predictable, common core beliefs defined by Dr Patrick Carnes[2] which almost every woman struggling with pornography will be able to identify in herself to some degree. These are:

1. I am a bad person, unworthy of love
2. No one will ever love me as I am
3. Sex is a necessity to feel good
4. My needs will never be met by anyone else.

Words women have shared with me as they describe themselves or how they feel include: worthless, ugly, disgusting, unlovable, unforgivable, irredeemable, too far gone, undesirable, unwanted, rejected, messy, alone, better off alone, desperate, bad, sinful, evil, undeserving and plenty more words which break my heart, and yet are far too familiar to my own voice many years ago. Many women even seek to punish themselves for their acting out or general state of being. This is in the form of self-harm, restriction of food or pleasures, or physical overexertion. I've even known women to think that anything that goes wrong (like tearing a favourite dress, a boring party, or hitting their elbow on a doorframe, etc.) is their fault and a deserved punishment.

Why would a woman believe these things about herself? Why would she pursue punishment, degrade herself and so firmly believe she is unworthy? Well, aside from the toxic culture women live in—where we are bombarded with sexualized media and products concocted to remind us we will never be as beautiful as the (photoshopped) model—plus the boatloads of shame that emanate from habitual and escalating porn use, many of these core beliefs are learned in childhood. Painful events and broken relationships such as the five outlined previously (family wounds, trauma, abandonment, loss, abuse) have a way of distorting a young or vulnerable person's perception.

When you're small, it is nearly impossible to understand that people can be mean, cruel and hurt you without it being your fault. The pain is new and confusing, and in order to explain and understand it the child takes it on and blames themselves. They must be 'bad', because why else would their parents, other adults or peers cause them harm? They don't have the capacity to understand that parents can be cruel, harmful or accidentally wound them. Internalising guilt is a child's way of understanding their situation, of making sense of a confusing environment.

Unfortunately, the weaponising of guilt and blame can further these beliefs, and ongoing pain only confirms a child's understanding of their unworthiness and how undeserving of nurturing intimacy they are. Children aren't the only ones who experience the distortion of positive self-perception. Adolescents, young adults and mature-aged women are all susceptible to the same blame game. Where there is pain and shame, there will be intrusive thoughts of unworthiness, guilt, and the unattainability of genuine intimacy. Uninterrupted, these become core beliefs which determine a woman's life choices and behaviours.

Core beliefs, although often extremely negative, can become comfortable. They are a familiar pair of glasses through which to see the world around you and understand yourself. If these beliefs are left undisturbed by truth, they become normal. The behaviours which stem from them become commonplace, and the piling up of shame from these behaviours goes unrecognised. This is especially true if your woundedness dates back to childhood or adolescence. It's just life, right? These core beliefs can become so ingrained that women have no idea they are actually carrying them around. The familiarity of a negative self-perception inhibits women from acknowledging an issue and getting the help they need to move forward and live a more abundant life. This is why it is so important to identify what core beliefs sustain your personal addiction tree. This is why we must reflect and dig deeper beneath the surface: to discover your roots. What may feel normal to you, may be unknowingly fuelling your addiction to pornography.

A woman struggling with pornography has an intimacy disorder. This stems from a specific or ongoing painful event, which left her feeling shame. In response to this distress, she seeks to explain the event by internalising guilt. The final outcome of this process is a woman's certainty that she is worthless. She believes 'I am worthless, no one could love me as I am, but I need sex to feel something good! Since I am so terrible, no one will willingly give me this—so I'll take care of it on my own'.

Look at this statement. Look at each of the four core beliefs. Do they resonate with you?

Has anyone implied or told you any of these things before? Why do you believe them?

Our core beliefs are formed by our experience of the world, and both the joys and wounds we experience and internalise. They are our way of understanding the world we live in, and they are nurtured by the environment we stay in. Underneath every female porn addict, is a woman with an intimacy disorder, who has known great pain and holds onto false core beliefs that continue this compounding cycle of addiction and shame. The only way to heal is to transform our fundamental beliefs about ourselves, our world and those around us. This is no easy task, but with a professional therapist, great support community and loads of self-care, this is entirely possible and will make all the difference in your recovery.

Conclusion

As you finish this chapter, I salute you. This may have been a haphazard journey through a land-mined warzone for you. It may have aroused feelings of pain you've been hiding from for a long time. This information demands introspection and an honest acknowledgement of your pain. We may have touched on all of the tender and frightened parts of you, or perhaps we prodded an angry heart. Whatever your experience, know that I'm proud of you and you've reached the end of this chapter! Give yourself some rest, take a nap, have a big fat cry if you need.

I hope you will take this opportunity to see the bigger picture of your porn problem. I hope your eyes have been taken off the shiny, distracting fruit and can see that your real issue is in fact your desperate search for intimacy, not sex. I hope you have been able to identify the pain you've been running from, or completely unaware of, so you can begin to deal with it in healing ways. May you take this chance to acknowledge what you really want—to be desired, affirmed and loved—and to identify what core beliefs fuel your lifestyle. It is my hope that after reading this chapter, you will be transformed from a woman who is only focused on eradicating porn behaviours, and who wants to blame others for her lack of recovery, into someone who is willing to reflect on her heart, and work on those inner wounds with professional support. I want you to become a recovery warrior—and I know you will.

Action Steps:

1. **Spend time journaling your answers to the reflection questions mentioned in this chapter.**
2. **Download, print out or draw your own addiction tree and personalise it. Using your own words, identify how each section of the tree manifests in your life. You can download the addiction tree from The Grace Spot, under the heading 'Get Help' followed by 'Download Worksheets' which you'll find under the 'Read my Book' section or at thegracespot.com/Restored-worksheets.**
3. **Chapter five spoke about triggers and their role in the addiction cycle. With the information from the tree analogy, can you identify any more personal pain triggers? Add them to your personalised diagram of the addiction cycle.**

CHAPTER SEVEN: WHAT NOW?

HEALING YOUR PAIN

That last chapter was tough. I know the first time I went through reflection on my underlying woundedness, it felt like performing open heart surgery on myself. Without anaesthetic. Can you relate? Digging into the whys and hows of your intimacy disorder may have triggered feelings of shame, anger, sadness or regret. As ironic as it seems, some women may even have been triggered to go and act out. Why? Because it hurts. After years of running and hiding from the reality of your broken heart, turning to face it head-on can be shattering. It feels like the protective bubble you've been living in suddenly bursts and, without porn there to comfort you and take you away from reality, where does that leave you? What do you do now?

That's exactly what this chapter is all about. I'm not going to dump a painful truth bomb on you and leave you hanging. Simply identifying issues isn't going to heal you. At this point, you have two choices: You can return to the familiarity of stuffing pain down inside and continue to live in denial of these truths (and probably get angry at me for even trying to bring it up), or you can learn how to be present in your pain, how to gently wade through the muck of the past and move forward into freedom.

I know it's tempting to ignore the pain of the past. It can feel like pandora's box; you fear if you start to let one little thing out, suddenly you'll be swamped in unbearable misery. I'll be honest with you: repressing your pain is the easier option. I mean, who really wants to uproot old hurts and do the dirty work of revisiting trauma? But ignoring it will not lead to the freedom you desire.

The healing that comes from acknowledging your pain is magnificent, but the journey is tough. You may have spent your life fleeing from the reality of your past. You may be anxious to drag other people into your mess. It's okay to be scared, and to feel a little lost. Remember, this is not about perfection. Recovery is about taking it at your own pace, and feeling safe and supported throughout the journey. Take as many cry breaks as you need. But you owe it to yourself to know what's truly going on. You've lived through such heart-ache, you're strong enough to feel a little more before the light comes pouring in. The awareness that comes from sitting with your pain has great power to break rituals and cycles. By letting the pain out in a safe way, you can take back control and power over your body and mind.

So, are you ready? Let's start with where your emotions are right now. Can you identify what you are feeling? Perhaps take some time to journal your thoughts and fears, or express yourself in whatever way suits you. If you're anything like me, you may be feeling overwhelmed. What do I do with all this pain? What on earth is going to come up if I just open the door a crack? How do I deal with this distress? Especially without porn?! You also may be feeling some bravery too. Is there just a part of you (or more!) that is curious to begin this journey? Are you somewhat excited to learn what really makes you tick, and deal with that? Are you hopeful you can feel more whole? Do you feel the time is right to try something different? I hope so. But if not, that's okay too. As you see results, I'm sure more of that brave curiosity will come.

Whatever you're feeling, this chapter is built to answer the 'What now?' question that inevitably follows a dump of painful reality. I'm hoping the following information will be a practical bite that brings hope after an intense chapter on intimacy and pain. I dearly hope this brings some calm, and a clear way forward.

I'm going to be sharing some activities and practices that can help to ground, affirm and direct you on this journey. These practices, along with others have the power to transform you from frightened apprehension into someone empowered and responsible, with tools to keep you grounded in reality without the need to escape using sex.

Now you're aware, you're responsible

Balance is a notoriously difficult task for addicted women. Does that resonate? We're often fighting against an all-or-nothing attitude and have a tendency to either dispose of all responsibility and blame others, or take on so much responsibility our backs and hearts are breaking. Where do you fall? Or perhaps you're a pendulum swinger as I am.

When it comes to recovery, balance is a skill you'll have to learn. Especially when it comes to personal responsibility. This was discussed as early as chapter two; do you remember? We discussed accountability. Your chosen accountability partner is there to walk with you, but in the end, you are responsible for your recovery. You must be honest with yourself, and them, and fulfil the expectations you discussed together.

That truth remains when it comes to your pain.

Now you are aware (or at least beginning to become aware) of your unique pain, you have a responsibility to deal with it.

You know you have an intimacy disorder. You know what triggers you. You know how addiction works in the brain and the points where you must break the ritual. You know your unique pains, and how they affect you to act out. Of course, you are only just beginning this journey and you will grow in awareness. You're not expected to know it all immediately. But to the best of your awareness, ability and knowledge—you are responsible. For example, if you know walking through the lingerie section at the store triggers you to act out, avoid it at all costs. If you know you're tempted to act out with an old sexual partner, cut off all contact. No amount of external support can make these decisions for you. They exist to support you on your personal journey and offer wisdom—which you are free to take or not.

Likewise, you are responsible for your pain. You are NOT in any way responsible for what happened to you, though. If you were hurt, abused, abandoned or taken advantage of in any way—*you are not responsible*. The responsibility for that lies directly on the abuser's head. However, you are responsible for what you do with that pain. Blaming the perpetrator can't heal you. Now that you are aware of your pain, you are responsible for your present and future actions.

It sucks, I know. It's unfair. Honestly, I wish I could go back in time and punch that ex-boyfriend in the face so hard it would reverse time and erase all the abuse and trauma he caused me. But it's not possible. And living in that fantasy can only keep me trapped in a cycle of anger and shame. He is responsible for harming me. He is the cause of my pain. He is accountable for what he did. However, I owned my responsibility to make wise choices going into the future. I was personally responsible for pursuing my recovery.

Again, you are NOT responsible for abuse. You are NOT responsible for actions which were out of your control. You are NOT responsible, even if someone told you so. Taking responsibility for your recovery and moving forward does NOT mean the person (or people) who harmed you are abdicated of their responsibility. It does NOT mean you are ignoring the event, sweeping it under the rug or forgetting. It doesn't even mean forgiveness. It just means you're taking your courage and choosing to flourish, despite what they did to you. It means all the energy spent looking back into the past can be thrown into forward motion, so you can experience freedom rather than a sore neck from looking behind you every day. We can only pray that, one day, those who harmed us will take responsibility for their actions and make amends too.

What steps do you take to deal with this pain?

Back to what on earth to do with all this new information. The following list isn't exhaustive by any means, it is simply a combination of healing practices I personally utilised in my own recovery, methods I discovered later in life, and practices suggested by fellow recovering women, some of which I still use today.

No two women are the same, so you'll find the practices that suit you best, and you may even find things outside of this recommendation list that work.

1. *Therapy*

You may have once thought 'I can do this alone!'.

Or perhaps you hoped you could keep this little secret just between you and one other person in the world.

Having one great friend or mentor to support you is amazing, and you may reach a healthy level of freedom. However, the saying 'it takes a village to raise a child' can easily be substituted into recovery.

It takes a village to support a healing woman.

It's more than likely you need professional therapy or counselling. Accountability is vital to your recovery, but your friend or mentor probably isn't equipped (nor has the time or mental space needed) to deal with serious mental health concerns. As much as she loves you, wants to fix all your problems and be there for you through the pain, it is unreasonable to expect that level of care.

Your accountability partner and other friends will be an invaluable source of comfort. You can share openly with them and be honest, but it takes a professional to walk through trauma and addiction. The bulk of your inner wound work must be done in a safe and professional environment.

There is no shame in seeking professional help. In fact, it's one of the bravest and wisest choices a woman can make. Reaching out for help is your first step; in the weeks, months or even years that come, you will need to be vulnerable, honest and committed. It's tough, but trust me, if you stick around long enough, you will feel better for it.

If you feel scared and overwhelmed, that's normal, but try to remember these things:

- Therapy is a proven method to heal woundedness.

- Therapists are trained to handle trauma and personal grief.
- Your therapist will help you develop insights and coping skills.
- A good therapist will never judge you. They've heard it ALL—don't feel ashamed. There will be no interruptions or story-topping. They are there to listen to you.
- Saying things out loud helps you understand them in a different way. This is an opportunity for an hour of guilt free venting.
- Therapists exist solely to explore personal pain, stress and trauma. They are invested in your healing.
- They are available as a crisis service, as well as for long term restoration.

These are indicators of a good therapist, which is most of them! However, if your therapist doesn't adhere to these general guidelines, or actively shames or reacts negatively towards you, you very well may need to find someone new to work with. If a therapist makes you feel uneasy (beyond the natural unease of pouring your heart out to a stranger), or dismisses your addiction or religious values, you have permission to leave. Leave, but seek another therapist.

Similarly, if your therapist is perfectly well behaved and good-intentioned but you just don't 'gel' with them, it's totally fine to look into another therapist. The relationship between a therapist and client is sacred, and you must feel safe and comfortable sharing. Some personalities just don't meld well. This person will be your healing guide, it's important to get this relationship right!

As a woman struggling with sexual issues, I found it important to see female psychologists and counsellors over the years. This made me feel safe, and prevented any inappropriate attachments forming with men on my end. Do your research when seeking a counsellor; read therapist's biographies (often listed on their website), read reviews or ask for recommendations from those previously in therapy. If you can, find someone who specialises in sexual addiction and trauma. If this is not available to you, professionals who have experience with eating disorders or other compulsive behaviours would be suitable as well. If you're a Christian, it can help to partner with someone with similar spiritual values, too. Your local mental health services may be limited, but the joy of the digital age is video-therapy! You may be able to access a specialist therapist through online video meetings. Do some research and see what's available. In saying all of this, most psychologists will be more than able to work with you and help you find healing, so if you are unable to find a specialist therapist online or locally, have no fear!

Therapy benefits even the most balanced, functional of women and their relationships. It is incredibly helpful to have an outside perspective, a listening ear and someone who has the training to move you towards a positive future. It is even more vital for women who feel stuck in addiction and deep in shame. I recommend any woman struggling with intimacy, porn, sex or compulsive masturbation book in with a therapist as soon as possible.

2. *Grieve*

Grieving isn't exclusive to death. You have permission and encouragement to grieve what you've lost, to mourn for your personal pain and the ways in which you were harmed or abandoned. Lament your fall into addiction, allow yourself to feel rightfully disappointed and sad about the events of your life which sting.

Grieving is an important part of recovery. Grieving means you travel through the motions of pain, anger, confusion, acceptance and healing.

Everyone has a unique way of grieving, but there are four predictable stages of grief you can expect as you reflect on your addiction and the wounds of the past. These are presented by Marnie Ferree in her landmark book *No Stones*[1].

- **Numbness:**

This is shock. A woman faced with pain or trauma will shut down, and function on auto-pilot. It is a state of semi-awareness and conscious or unconscious denial. This is the initial stage, when pain is too overwhelming to feel. Numbness 'protects' us from having to feel.

- **Yearning/Searching**:

This is deep longing for what you lost. You yearn for a person or thing. It feels like a gaping hole in your heart, a black hole that sucks the joy out of everything. You search without success for whatever it is you miss so deeply. It may feel like part of you is missing. Without that person, that event, that nurturing or touch in your life, you feel void. This is the unique horror of grief; the chilling awareness of loss. This stage is characterised by deep depression and sadness. You may find yourself looking back at the painful event and asking 'Why?' …

'What if?'. It feels unjust, and much energy is spent grieving that missing piece of the puzzle.

- **Disorganisation**:

The realization dawns: Life as you know it will never be the same. You are getting closer to acceptance and jumping off the hamster wheel of grief, but questions disorient you. You may ask 'Who am I now? What is my purpose? How do I go on?'. You may wonder how you will actually heal in light of this uncovered trauma or pain. How will you put the jumbled pieces back together? Is it possible to live a normal life? This is an awareness that you were wronged, that something isn't right … you want to heal, but how? Life is chaos and confusion. You feel lost and overwhelmed. This stage is characterised by anger.

- **Reorganisation**:

Acceptance. Coming to terms with the loss. This stage brings the ability to experience pain and painful memories without being overwhelmed. Although scarred, a woman who reaches this stage believes life can go on and she can find some meaning despite the mess. Reorganisation is renewal or restoration. Out of chaos comes order. You may feel more confident in naming and taming your demons, without the need to medicate.

As Ferree says, these stages aren't clear cut, and women may well leapfrog through them, return to previous steps, experience multiple stages at once, and cycle through this process a number of times before feeling free of the grief. It develops and changes over time along with the unique circumstances of life. Honestly, it's a mess, but if you examine the chaos that arises, you will be able to identify the different stages and where you might be at in the journey. I wish it was simpler, but healing never is.

There is no time limit on healing, either. There's no rush. It takes as long as it takes, and the grieving process lasts as long as it needs to. If the sorrow of grief holds on for an exceptionally long time, it may be an indicator that something needs to change in your overall recovery process. Re-evaluate and ask your accountability partner or therapist if they can identify an area in which you need to pursue change. But sometimes you can be doing all you can, and still grieve. This is okay. Let it be.

Grieving hurts, but allowing yourself to feel everything that comes along with it is beginning the journey to acceptance. If you allow the grief cycle to occur, you can finally be released from its pain. It is a difficult but necessary process. You have permission to grieve the wounds of the past.

3. *Inner Child Work*

Most women with intimacy issues have pain that reaches all the way back to childhood. The recovering woman still has a hurt and frightened little girl within. Do you feel her? Can you sense her pain? Or have you hardened your heart to her by ignoring her cries and calling them weak?

You cannot change the past, but as a grown woman you are now capable of acknowledging the little girl's pain, of nurturing her, comforting her and giving her as much love as she needs. You are in a place where you can look back and acknowledge what she needed, and what was taken from her. Give her a safe place to cry, let her grieve, be vulnerable and allow her to name her pain.

Think back to your childhood:

- What needs did you have that were not met?

- Did you lose your childhood?
- What words did you need to hear but didn't?
- Did you feel abandoned? How?
- Was anything taken from you?
- Did you have to be a surrogate spouse?
- What was unfair about your upbringing?
- If you could recreate your childhood what would it look like?
- Did you miss out on security, nurturing, comfort, physical touch or dignity?
- Did you get enough play?
- Is your inner child frightened?
- Was your inner child shut down or told not to feel?
- Were you abused or hurt growing up?
- Are you keeping any secrets from your childhood?

Did any of these reflections bring up strong feelings? No matter the time and distance from our childhood, that little wounded girl is within us, begging for attention and love.

If you grew up in an unsafe or less healthy family, accessing and nurturing your inner child may be difficult. It may feel foreign; like talking to a ghost. If you have little, or a distorted, experience of adult care towards children, you may feel you don't have anything to replicate. How do you reconnect with that little girl crying in her room? How do you fulfil her needs when you've never experienced nurturing yourself? It's not always simple, but trust yourself. If you went without as a child, it's likely you know in your heart what you need. The things that felt unjust, unfair and painful were exactly that, so lavish upon your inner child the opposite of these negative experiences. Does she feel void of affirmation? Play? Independence? Was she put down and bullied? Did she carry the burdens of her parents? What is it that you always craved in your heart of hearts? As a child, what did you desire that would take away the pain? If you still struggle to connect with the inner girl, why not think of another child? It could be a niece or nephew, the child of a friend or a random baby rolling by in a pram! If that child was hurting or in danger, what would you do? How would you speak to them, touch them and show love? This may help you to connect with your own Inner Child needs.

This is very deep work which can unearth repressed memories and pain, so please make sure you're surrounding yourself with support, including that of a professional therapist or counsellor. It is possible to trigger yourself into a relapse when attempting to heal if you're doing it alone.

To finish our discussion on Inner Child work, here are a few practical suggestions for sending some love and care to that little girl inside. These are based on Ferree's detailed instructions on Inner Child work in *No Stones*[1].

- Buy a soft toy.

I'm serious, take an afternoon to go shopping and pick out your ideal cuddly buddy! I don't care how old, professional, cool or uncertain you are—we are never too old for physical comfort. Pick a stuffed toy that appeals to you. It may be soft and tiny enough to fit in your hand, or it might be a big cuddly teddy bear. Maybe you need a dragon or lion to protect you. I have a toy sloth that gives me comfort when I'm home alone, sick or away from my husband. There is something cathartic and safe about holding onto a fluffy, soft toy—especially at night when fear can creep in.

- Let her cry.

Weep for every little loss you suffered. Nothing is too small to feel. If you weren't allowed to show emotion as a child, let it out now.

- Keep her safe.

Inner Child work is deeply emotional, and cannot be done while in survival mode. Do not attempt to probe this deeply if you are not in a space where you have support and safety.

- Connect your pain to a specific age.

What's your earliest memory of pain? Find a picture of yourself at that age and speak comforting words to it (yeah, it feels weird at first, but give it a try!).

- What did you wish you heard as a child?

'I love you!' 'You are precious' 'You are so funny!' 'No matter what I'll protect you'? Discover what you missed out on, and practice daily affirmations using that childhood picture.

- Play.

A lot of us missed out on play as children. I know it may feel weird as a grown woman, but pursue what you missed out on! Visit a lolly shop, the zoo, have a sleepover, play old video games, draw with chalk, skip or go to a trampoline park. Grab a sister in recovery or a close friend and have some real fun! You deserve it.

4. *Mindfulness and Grounding Practices*

Mindfulness is hard! Have you ever sat down on a yoga mat to meditate with all the best intentions in the world of connecting with your inner self, only to find your mind wandering further than you've physically walked in months?

Have you ever experienced a total melt-down triggered by something seemingly insignificant, or found negative thoughts cascading all over your day and paralysing you? You're not alone, trust me. Far too often, I've found my own mind wandering into the distance despite trying to ground myself. I've frequently let shame rule my behaviours, rather than careful mindfulness. I've cried into more than one bowl of ice-cream and splurged on online shopping like a mad-woman to try to quieten the tornado of red-hot emotion in my head. But I know there is value in practicing mindfulness and grounding techniques; I am practicing them and learning right beside you.

Obviously, I'm not a mindfulness guru (I'm probably more of a mindless one), but I know first-hand just how quickly our minds can spiral out of control. As an addict, or someone with compulsive behaviours, this is a dangerous reality. Mindfulness is an important skill to develop as you heal; it is one of the best practices for dealing with immediate pain and strong emotions, not just for addicts but any woman!

So, what *is* mindfulness anyway? You may be picturing yourself sitting on a yoga mat, surrounded by incense and completely erasing all thoughts. That might do it for some folk, but the kind of mindfulness I'm advocating isn't about having a blank mind or reaching enlightenment. It's also not limited to a specific time or place; it's not something you decide to do for thirty minutes a week then forget. The type of mindfulness a recovering woman needs is constant and ever-accessible; it is available at any given moment of stress or trigger. Mindfulness in this context simply means taking the time to compassionately and gently identify and acknowledge your emotions, thoughts and actions.

Mindfulness is acknowledging what emotion you feel in the moment, without attaching shame, expectation or judgement to it. This is difficult, as we are so used to placing moral values on what we feel. For example, being sexually triggered and feeling rejected or hurt are often laden with shame. We judge ourselves for feeling or reacting in these ways. Do these inner statements sound familiar?

'You shouldn't feel upset, it's not even a big deal.'

'You're so weak/pathetic.'

'What's wrong with you?!'

'You're so stupid/disgusting!'

One emotion easily tumbles into another, and soon enough you've snowballed into an emotional crash or acting out. It is difficult to experience painful emotions, but remember, feelings are okay. In times of high emotion, your old habit of anaesthetising pain or discomfort with porn might rock up to say 'hello!'. This is your familiar reaction to feeling. Women like to 'numb out' or try to feel something euphoric instead of hurtful. Fair enough! Learning to sit with your discomfort and allowing your emotions to ebb and flow can keep acting out at bay. Mindfulness not only helps you understand yourself better (by actually engaging with your emotions, instead of numbing out or escaping) but is a practice that has the power to halt addictive behaviours.

As you've been examining your history and wounded behaviours, have you felt strong emotions arise? Did they seem to multiply the more thought you gave them? Did your emotions spiral out of control leaving you feeling helpless and messy?

To ease the chaos, practice identifying your primary emotion, feeling or thought, right from the beginning; describe and acknowledge how you feel, in the same way you might describe a painting on the wall, or a piece of furniture in the room. You might like to think of it as capturing it—this even ties in nicely with some biblical wisdom (*We take captive every thought to make it obedient to Christ.* 1 Corinthians 10:5). Do this before the thought runs wild by simply naming and owning it. You may need to repeat the acknowledgement in your head (or out loud) a few times to keep the spiral at bay and remain grounded in reality. Keep acknowledging what's actually going on for you without running wild with it, and without attaching shame or judgement.

For example, you might acknowledge 'I feel rejected, and my feelings are hurt' or 'I feel anxious, I'm worried people won't like me' or 'I was triggered by a sexual image, I am aroused and want to act out'.

Sit with that statement and let it be. No judgement. No shame. No explanation or diving off into fantasy. You are entitled to feel. There are no moral attachments to emotions. No good or bad. If you start to think 'I shouldn't feel that', stop; take a breath and tell yourself that it doesn't matter whether I should or shouldn't; this is what I do feel right now. I know it's hard—you're used to being pretty critical on yourself and your emotions and other people have probably given you negative input too. Mindfulness takes radical self-compassion and love in the moment we think we deserve it least.

Mindfulness is about staying present. It is grounding yourself in reality when fantasy wants to take you away to a 'better place'. When emotions hit or something visually triggers you, try to stay in the present moment by speaking to yourself (in your head or out loud). It could be a prayer, Bible passage, a funny statement, you could describe everything you're seeing or doing, or sing a song. You may use a physical reminder, something you can hold onto or look at in times of temptation. Anything that keeps you where your feet are planted. What are some ideas you can use in your journey?

5. *Discover your emotional needs and meet them without sex.*

You'd be correct in saying we want to distance ourselves from fantasy-land, and not give too much of our attention to that magical place where nothing is real and we lose track of reality. However, when it comes to the hefty work of healing and working through the pain that fuels your addiction, there's a time and a place—and a way—to use your fantasies to your advantage. They can help you heal!

What?!

Let me tell you how my accountability partner and I did this. Before anything else, Mel and I made sure we had a solid foundation of honesty and regularity before we moved from our basic accountability to recovery work. When we both had some decent sobriety, and improved coping mechanisms (read: not sprinting to porn or masturbation the moment life got difficult), we began the next phase of our journey. For us, it was about six months into regular accountability. You'll know when you're ready.

Together, we reflected on and discussed the nature of our most common fantasies. We didn't share the gory sexual details or dwell on the feelings they aroused but spoke in general, non-triggering terms. We used five questions inspired by Ferree to help us get curious about what lay behind these fantasies of ours.

1. What is my most common fantasy?
2. Who is involved and who may they represent?
3. What is the setting?
4. What is happening?
5. What do you think the emotional need behind the fantasy is?

Fantasies are a window into the soul. They have the power to reveal and help you understand your deepest emotional desires and needs that have gone unmet. Fantasies can give you valuable insight into wounds you subconsciously carry. Why is this?

The world you create in your mind represents your ideal existence. When reality becomes overbearing, fantasy-land is a safe place to visit. It soothes the pain of existence; it is a place where you are one hundred percent in control, and absolutely anything is possible. It is a secret place where your deepest desires can be manifested. It can feel like the only safe place to be vulnerable enough to express what a woman truly wants in life. It's a place where you can be anything you want: rich, famous, cherished, desired and powerful. If you could snap your fingers and make your favourite fantasy come true, would you? I know I would. It may not turn out so successful in reality, but your heart craves it.

Mel and I had both experienced a range of pains, losses and trauma in our lives. We experienced feelings of being unworthy, unloved and unwanted. Probably our most common wound was that of feeling out of control; events of the past had left us feeling powerless over what happened to our bodies and lives.

Thus, it was no surprise that our most common fantasies centred around being in control, and being cherished.

These fantasies were our minds way of coping. If we couldn't get what we needed in reality (or, hadn't in the past), we would create a new realm in our heads where we could access these needs. I mean, it's pretty ingenious of our brains to look out for us in that way. But in the end, fantasy only keeps you locked inside the trauma. When you re-enter reality, it still hurts. Genuine healing comes when you can identify and deal with the pains and emotional needs associated with that fantasy. Once you identify your unmet needs and wounds, you can work on finding ways to have those needs met without compulsive sexual behaviour or other harmful actions. Many of our emotional needs can be met through non-sexual relationships such as family, friends, mentors and even pets. It's easy to forget this in a sex-saturated world, especially when you've been seeking all your answers in pornography.

It's likely you have a number of common fantasies you cycle through; that's very normal. Women often struggle with multiple painful experiences over their lifetime. You may also come up with a number of different conclusions; emotions aren't often clear-cut! This is normal too. Allow yourself time to reflect and discuss your thoughts with your therapist or accountability partner. You might uncover a number of different fantasies, and it can take time to gain clarity on what they mean.

6. *Spiritual healing*

It is often in the darkest times that we can see God most clearly. His light shines bright in the night. When your heart aches, and your mind is spinning from the revelation of hidden pain, it can be hard to know where to turn for help and comfort. All of the previous recommendations are important for healing, but God is your most accessible source of comfort throughout all of this. He is present in every moment, and through every experience. And He cares. Head towards that light.

Chapter eight will deal with spiritual matters in much more detail, but for now, I want you to remember He is there, and He is for you. I know just how difficult it can feel to connect with Him after a lifetime of struggle. There are many reasons you may not feel able, or even want, to engage spiritually: shame, resentment, anger and spiritual abuse are just a few reasons. Perhaps you want to connect with Jesus but the example of the Church is just too much, and it pushes you away. Christianity (and Christians) can be awful. Of course, that's going to colour your view of God.

There is power in the spiritual, though.

So, I encourage you to forget anything unhelpful you've been taught about how to connect with God, and do it your way. Seek Him on your own terms. Prayer and spiritual connection don't have to look like being silent and bowing your head in Church—but it can. You might feel close to God in a number of other ways: running, dancing, reading theology books, singing, creating art, being in nature, expressing your anger towards Him (yes, you can swear at God), listening to worship music or any other number of activities. Do whatever you can to grow closer to God. He is the ultimate comforter and healer, and He can handle whatever you bring. He can give you the courage to face your pain head-on, and the stamina to walk through therapy, self-reflection and recovery work.

Personally, I have found there is so much power in music. This is why The Grace Spot has curated a playlist of healing music which is available through Spotify; simply log in and follow 'The Grace Spot: Healing Music' to access it. I find these songs to be incredibly moving, and act as prayers when I am overwhelmed and have no words or wisdom. They quieten my aching soul and help me to hear the Holy Spirit. They are a great and easy place to start re-connecting with God when your soul is weary and you seem to have forgotten how.

Conclusion

Did any of these tasks shout out to you? As you read, did your heart peep up a little and say 'Oh, I think I need that!'? Parts of you may have resisted. It's scary to consider bearing your all to a therapist or opening up the floodgates of Inner Child pain! But you probably know you must tackle it head on in order to get anywhere new. And you should feel empowered to do so; look how far you've come! Look how hard you've worked! You've got this in the bag, girl.

None of these practices on their own can heal you, they all take work, persistence and rely on the foundation you've created already: continued accountability, understanding your cycle, self-care, sobriety and facing your inner pain.

I hope this chapter provided you with some practical guidelines for when the pain becomes overwhelming. You don't have to do this alone, and there are tried and true ways to face and defeat the woundedness that fuels your addiction to porn. I hope you see a way forward from the pain of the past. I want you to know there's no short-cut or quick cure-all for addiction. But there is a pathway you can follow, and you can experience freedom and joy again. There are ways to deal with the pain, both short and long term, and I hope you'll pursue these methods. I'd like to encourage you to take the first practice seriously, and consider contacting a professional counsellor or psychologist to walk you through recovery. This book can give both you and your chosen accountability partner a guideline for recovery, but a therapist will be able to be present in your regular life, see you face to face and use their training and experience to take you deeper into healing. At this stage, you're at a point where you're facing the deeper stuff. You require more support than just accountability and helpful books and blogs. You need a diving partner to get into your soul.

Don't stop there, though—choose another practice and give it a go (with your support network).

As I mentioned before, recovery from addiction is a dual pathway. There's sobriety and then there's healing. The first part of this book focused on restricting your vice and reflecting on yourself and your addiction. These past two chapters have particularly focused on your underlying pain. And finally, as you may have guessed, the final chapters will focus on restoration. To recover, you must seek sobriety, you must examine pain and yourself, and then actively restore positivity to your life. There's no use delving into all this pain and just leaving it out on the kitchen sink to stink up the house! With a therapist, and some of these tools, you can begin to dismantle and dispose of it over time. And in the following chapters, we're going to discuss replacing that stinking mess with beauty. It's time to make a new life for yourself and replace that addiction tree with something that flourishes in joy, hope and positivity.

Action Steps:

1. **Spend some time journaling or creatively expressing your emotional reaction to this chapter.**

2. **Specifically identify and write down what emotions and memories have been stirred.**
3. **Identify and write down what you need to do to seek healing or further support (therapy, Inner Child work, grieve, mindfulness, spiritual healing, examination of fantasies, etc.).**
4. **Make a plan of action. How are you going to pursue healing? Be as specific as possible (e.g. call local counselling service and make appointment, buy soft toy and spend time with your inner child etc.).**

CHAPTER EIGHT: YOUR UNDERSTANDING OF GOD

I wish I could have seen your face when you first picked up this copy of *Restored*. When I consider the women who will purchase this book I imagine a great sense of relief upon their faces. *Finally, a book for female porn users!* It was always my aim that women who saw the title *Restored* would experience just a glimmer of hope and believe, even if just for a moment, that they themselves could be restored too. If the front cover of this book piqued your interest and empowered you enough to dedicate your time to reading it—and you're still here—I'm so glad!

However, I am well aware that despite the hopeful title of this guide, it may not feel super positive thus far. When is the restoring happening? you ask. All the talk about pain, trauma and addiction may have left you feeling like a dilapidated house being pulled down wall by wall. I've stripped away your protective layers and coping mechanisms, I've revealed your deepest pain and now you're just a bare house frame, exposed and barely standing. *Fun!* Right? This may not be easy or fun, but it is the first step towards restoration.

When you're rebuilding, you've got to pull down everything that once stood first, and then you begin to restore your home from the ground up. With a fresh foundation, it has the potential to be built into a strong, beautiful, unshakable home. Likewise, we're restoring your life. We're examining the foundations and framework and pulling down what's broken and weak, in order to replace it with something stronger and better.

I'm not working with you to simply destroy the life you have (even if it is less than ideal), but to gently pull down the damaged parts of you, all in order to help you rebuild and restore.

The restoration process began when you opened this book for the very first time. But right now, we're about to delve into the real nitty gritty of restoration and rebuilding your life, core beliefs and attitudes. And it all starts with God.

God equals … yikes?

How does that make you feel? What was your initial gut response when I mentioned that little three letter word? For many Christian women struggling with pornography, the idea of God provokes mixed emotions. Sometimes considering God results in fear, hatred, resentment, bitterness or emptiness. The way some women know God, or know of Him, is in terms of darkness and pain, while others may love the idea of an all-loving God but it all just feels inaccessible.

Still, there are women who hold onto God for dear life as they rollercoaster through addiction. He is their only certainty and hope in life, and He breathes life into their lungs day by day as they continue to choke on the toxic air of pornography.

Of course, for others the idea of God is fairly neutral. No big reaction occurred when they discovered they'd be examining their relationship with God today. He's just a vague part of life, so this process shouldn't be too difficult. Wherever you're at, we're starting the journey to restoring intimacy with God by examining your current relationship with Him, your beliefs and the emotions attached to thoughts of religion or faith. Even if you feel like you're in a swell place with God right now, it won't hurt to follow along as we reflect together. You never know what God may teach you.

Start at the beginning

Let's begin with some simple reflection. Ask yourself the following questions and do the activities listed and spend time thinking through your answers. You might like to journal this section.

1. How is your relationship with God?
2. What do you struggle with? (doubt, forgiveness, etc.)
3. Draw a picture of you and God. What do you think He's like? Ignore artistic quality, this is about how you perceive God and how you engage with Him.
4. What does the previous step reveal to you?
5. Do you believe you are worth loving? (Foremost by God, but also by others)
6. Has anything about God or your relationship with Him or the Church been on your mind lately? What is it?

Kat's Story

Kat participated in this reflection activity and shared some of her thoughts about her view of God and her pornography habit with me:

When the topic of 'God' came up, I had a gut-level negative reaction. To be honest, I rolled my eyes and thought about skipping over it but I figured 'what do I have to lose except feeling like crap?'. I tried it. My drawing of God and I was pretty revealing, actually. God was large and foreboding, I drew other people happily surrounding Him, but I was a small and distant figure in the picture. I drew myself and God in dark colours.

I was raised in a conservative Christian home, attended church throughout the week and knew the basics of Christianity. I was taught Jesus died on a cross to save me, because I was a sinner. I knew that lust was a sin and Jesus loved me.

When I was fourteen, I found porn on my dad's laptop. Being fairly sheltered, I was drawn in. I was curious about how these people were acting, and intrigued by the intensity. It was two weeks later I returned. From then on, surfing the web for pornography and erotic fiction became a regular habit. I continued going to church, but my heart began to feel more and more distant from God. I knew about all the love and grace stuff, but I just felt so especially dirty for what I was doing every day.

The thing that really broke my relationship with God was youth group. One evening, the topic was masturbation and sex. Part of me was afraid, but I was also secretly hopeful. Maybe I would get an opportunity to talk to one of the leaders about my struggle. With trepidation, I attended the event, only to come home broken and in tears.

They only addressed the boys. They specifically said 'we know girls don't really have this issue' (with porn, masturbation) but they kept us present so we could understand what the boys go through, so we could dress modestly around them and not tempt them.

To me, all I heard was 'women don't have this issue' or 'if they do, it's too bad and sinful to talk about'. My youth group leaders were my image of God, so I felt like God Himself was dismissing me and judging me for such a heinous unfeminine sin. I seriously felt too far gone for forgiveness.

I still believe in God, and I pray sometimes. But since then, I've really never felt close to God or felt anything spiritual—I just fake it and go through the motions at church. I always feel guilty and like there's a dark cloud over my head. I think I should talk to my counsellor about this, I hope she understands.

There are a thousand different things that can distort our view of God and get between us knowing intimacy and safety with Him. Pornography, habitual sin, false teaching, feeling unheard, alienated or being downright harmed by the Church are just some of the reasons people have given for feeling distant and irredeemable to God, despite having grown up in Christian homes. I know this breaks God's heart. I know there is intimacy in His arms, safety with Him, and boundless love and kindness to be poured out upon you.

I, too have been in the place of feeling shamed by dead religion and rules, feeling like forgiveness and mercy were undeserved and impossible. I lived my addicted life fleeing from God, and isolating myself from His people. Deep in my heart, I didn't believe I was lovable. Not by people, or God. He personally came and karate kicked that idea right out of my head, though. Through a process involving friends, prayer and incredible spiritual experiences (and a lot of ugly crying if we're being honest), He showed me undeniable love. He showed me I was worthy, and I didn't need to hide from Him. He saw it all and He still chose the cross. He truly, irrevocably loved me and always would.

The words contained in this chapter aren't just theology or theory to me, they're the fruit of my real-life experience with Jesus and religion, and include common themes shared with me by struggling women.

The following section will deal with four common experiences and beliefs about God, as experienced by women struggling with pornography. These are:

1. God isn't delivering me from my addiction. What gives?!
2. God couldn't love and forgive me.
3. God is distant, angry and wants to punish me.
4. I don't know what I believe anymore. I'm hurt and have doubts.

I'd like you to reflect on these statements. How true are they for you? When and why did you start believing them? Could they be distorted views of God, influenced by negative human experiences? How are these beliefs impacting your daily life, spiritually and emotionally? Are you happy to continue the way things are? Or could you envisage a future where God truly is love?

We'll be examining each of these belief patterns in detail; I hope you can open your heart and mind to alternative views of God, even if just for a moment.

I want you to read my words as gentle advice, not as words intended to rebuke, shame or act as an ultimatum regarding your personal faith. I have no claim to being totally right, I'm not God! But I am a woman who's known grace beyond belief, a woman who's walked in both worlds, with and without intimacy with God.

It's okay if you don't experience a heart-level spiritual transformation as you read this. I do not want this to be another opportunity for you to guilt or shame yourself for not being good enough or achieving enough. When it comes to religion, there's a lot of room for shame and shoulds. The Church has done enough of this, and I bet you've had enough of it from yourself, too. So, let's lay the shoulds and expectations aside for a while. Let's end the idea that you need to be transformed right now, by doing all the right things.

This is spiritual healing, and generally, it takes time. This may be the first step in that direction, or perhaps it will be part of a journey that is already happening for you. We can never force God's hand, but I know He wants to see you into healing and restoration. So why don't you stop and pray if you feel able to, ask God to lead you and reveal truths to you. Ask Him to open your heart and mind to new ideas, and allow yourself to fully feel what comes from these statements. This is another opportunity for healing, and to be completely honest with yourself. Don't stop after this chapter, keep coming back, and keep examining your view of God, and how other people may have impacted it. Examine the Bible and pray to Jesus to seek truth, and don't simply feed on your pastor, the internet or even what I'm throwing to you. Learn to live this yourself.

1. God isn't delivering me from my addiction. What gives?!

Christians sing about God 'breaking chains' *a lot*. It all sounds very instantaneous and intense, but most people aren't instantly delivered from their addiction through prayer or spiritual means alone.

Have you prayed about your addiction too many times to count? Does the desperate cry 'God, please deliver me! I'll do anything you want if you take my desire away' sound familiar? Or perhaps it was once a regular request but is now a distant memory. He never came through.

This is understandably frustrating. If God wants you to live in purity and freedom, why isn't He making that possible? Why is He ignoring you? It doesn't make sense. At this point, women tend to decide that either God, or they themselves, are fundamentally at fault and flawed.

But what if we've got it all wrong? What if true healing came from overcoming all the obstacles on the journey *alongside* God, rather than clicking our fingers and getting whisked away from all the pain? What if, instead of suddenly breaking the chains for us, God chooses to give us the *tools* to break free from those chains? What if He provides the directions to slowly crush those links instead of doing it all without us? What if He wants to teach us something through the process?

If God delivered all of us immediately, we would miss out on so much. Sure, it would be easier, but have you considered what you may not gain if you didn't have to work at recovery? Consider courage, vulnerability or the intimacy that grows between friends and spouses when they're truly honest with each other. What about the false beliefs and lies that live within us from childhood or abuse? These would never be uncovered and exposed for their lies if we didn't have to dig. Our souls and minds would never truly heal, we'd simply have part of us removed.

The often long and slow recovery process is a redemptive gift from God. The season may be long and hard, but it is brimming with valuable lessons and insight. When frustration strikes, remember the words of James 1:2-4:

Consider it pure joy, my brothers and sisters, whenever you face trials of many kinds, because you know that the testing of your faith produces perseverance. Let perseverance finish its work so that you may be mature and complete, not lacking anything. If any of you lacks wisdom, you should ask God, who gives generously to all without finding fault, and it will be given to you.

God is working to make you mature and complete, and sometimes that comes through trials of many kinds.

Continue to pray, though. Instantaneous deliverance from addiction is possible, but it's not common. Shannon is one of the women who did experience such an immediate deliverance from her addiction. She contacted me through Facebook and shared her story with me.

After struggling with porn, masturbation and empty sexual encounters for many years, she repeated the sinner's prayer and found sexually explicit material made her physically ill from then on. She is now living in freedom from those unwanted sexual behaviours. In His wisdom, God knew Shannon needed this, and He knows what you need as well. There is no cookie-cutter recovery model when it comes to God. So ask Him for freedom, but if you find yourself continuing to struggle, why not pray for courage for the journey, too? Pray for insight into your heart and what needs to be healed. If you're married, pray for your spouses' healing and a better relationship. Talk to God about how you feel and the pain you've experienced. In doing this, you deepen your relationship with God, and acknowledge the need for more than simply stopping the behaviour, but a deeper, long-lasting recovery.

God isn't withholding freedom from you because of a lack of faith or worthiness or because He's on a wicked power-trip. Rather, He's inviting you on a journey. God sees the amazing healing and growth that lies ahead of you; He wants to see you uproot toxic beliefs and memories; He wants to walk with you as you replant your life in nourishing soil; He wants you to learn to relate to Him every day, not only for a once off request. I believe He wants to raise up many women who have walked the whole walk, who can then minister to others who are struggling with shame and porn and feel completely alone like you once did. God has a plan mapped out for you, and even though it's going to be painful and long, you can trust He has your best interests at heart. It's almost impossible to comprehend in the moment, but the recovery journey, rather than immediate deliverance, is actually the greater gift.

2. God couldn't love and forgive me.

Addiction thrives in the dark. With no outside input, shame flourishes. Shame is different to guilt. Guilt is the feeling of knowing you've done something wrong. Usually, it leads to repentance, apology and forgiveness. Shame, however, is guilt gone rogue. It is a poison that eats you up from the inside. Shame takes the feeling of having done something wrong, and transposes it upon your self. Instead of doing something wrong, you become the thing that is wrong. Shame is the belief that you are flawed, bad, wrong and unlovable.

When you believe you are fundamentally flawed and wrong—women have used the term 'freak' or 'disgusting' to describe themselves to me—it is easy to see how the belief that 'God couldn't love or forgive me' sneaks in. A woman full to the brim with shame feels unworthy of forgiveness and love; she doesn't consider forgiveness and acceptance achievable in her human relationships, let alone with the great God of the universe! She isolates herself from Christian community (what if they found out?!) as well as from God Himself.

Do you feel 'too far gone' for forgiveness and love? Have you learned that you have to earn your forgiveness and love from authority figures? Do you 'make up' for your sins by serving extra hard at church, or helping others to your own detriment? Are porn splurges followed by rigid rule keeping and intense Christian service to the point of exhaustion?

If the belief 'God couldn't love and forgive me' resonates with you, why do you think that is? Is this the character of the God of the Bible?

I suggest not. If you've been taught that forgiveness has a limit, or love must be earned by good behaviour, I urge you to spend time with Jesus, to read the New Testament and chat to someone who seems to know a wholeness and fullness of life in Christ. I'd also like to introduce you to a few historical figures which serve to me as evidence that unconditional love and forgiveness are available in full, to all people, at any time, from this moment forward!

King David

King David is proof to me that you can be sinful, sexually compulsive and manipulative at the same time as being chosen, loved and influentially used by God. Feels wrong to say that, doesn't it? Obviously, I think God wants us to avoid the sinful crap, but even when we don't it doesn't change His love for us. His forgiveness is everlasting. Being adored by God isn't reserved only for those 'perfect Christian women'. Have you ever met one of these rare creatures? Me neither.

Let's talk about King David. He features in, and contributed to, a number of books within the Bible. He is often held up as the portrait of a godly leader and most Christians and non-Christians are familiar with his name. Oh, and did I mention he was the great, great, great (times about forty-one) granddaddy of Jesus? What an honour! And yet his sin is infamous. You know the one.

2 Samuel 11 depicts the event. David, standing on his rooftop, sees a woman bathing. (This wasn't the suburban lifestyle we know today, during this time roofs were flat and people washed there). She is beautiful, and

his lust is piqued. Being the king, he childishly demands information (think, an ancient style Facebook stalk), which reveals she is a married woman. He knows her husband, he is fighting enemies for David at that very moment, in the war the king was meant to be leading (his sin didn't start with Bathsheba, it began when he shrugged off his responsibilities). Despite the husband situation, David uses his kingly powers to summon the woman and have sex with her. No mention of consent, either. He saw, he liked, he got what he wanted. She later becomes pregnant from this encounter, and good old King D freaks out and has her hubby killed on the battlefield. What a jerk!

And yet, he is forgiven. He goes on to lead Israel into their most prosperous years and shares an intimate relationship with God as seen in the psalms. In fact, if you turn to Psalm 51 (a favourite for recovering women) you can see his intimate and vulnerable cry for forgiveness and purity of heart. He confidently seeks forgiveness for his sins and offers his whole heart to the Lord, rather than fleeing or hiding from Him in silence. And we see the fruit of this as the Bible story continues. He isn't cut off from God's Spirit or affections, but called a 'man after God's own heart' (Acts 13:22). His messiness and sexual turmoil do not exclude him from either salvation or an on-the-ground relationship with the Lord of all.

David was a great king; he was faithful and knew God intimately. He was also a sexual being with desires that sometimes ran rampant. Because of grace, these two things can exist together. Remember this next time you try to cut yourself off from God after a lapse.

Hosea's wife (Gomer)

The book of Hosea reveals a very telling tale of God's unconditional and patient love for all people. Gomer is a prostitute, a woman excluded from society and looked down upon. There is no telling how many sexual encounters she had, nor how degrading they were. And yet, this is the woman God chooses to reveal His love through. If you haven't read this short book, I recommend you do. It's powerful. Short story even shorter though, God commands a prophet by the name of Hosea to marry this prostitute and show her love.

In the Old Testament God used images or symbols to speak to people. Prophecy was often dramatic and visual, and this event is an example of this. Hosea represented God, and Gomer represented Israel. During their marriage, the Bible tells us how she was continually unfaithful and fled back to her life of sexual sin. Yet God continued to command Hosea to take her back, love, clothe and provide for her. He was to love her unconditionally, no matter how many times she turned away from his love and kindness.

This real-life analogy was speaking to Israel, and the sexual unfaithfulness of Gomer represented their many sins and unfaithfulness to Yahweh. It wasn't necessarily sexual sin for them—it was predominantly idol worship which drew them away from their kind and generous God. God was saying, I love you! I will always be here to take you back! I will forgive you! I won't abandon or forsake you, even if you turn away and spit in my face! I'll be waiting, my children!

That message remains for you today, sister. I absolutely love this story. When I first read the book of Hosea, I was stunned. I related so much to this degraded woman, I felt like my sexual struggles identified me, I felt like an unfaithful and dirty woman and I believed I would be abandoned. I was unlovable. Yet it says the opposite. It says I am welcomed back into my Father's arms. So great is His love for us, that He is a patient and generous husband taking back an unfaithful wife over and over again.

Rahab

Rahab was a prostitute; she had a long list of lovers and possibly experienced social ostracising and shame. She did not live a holy or pleasant life, nor was she one of God's chosen people, an Israelite. Imagine meeting an atheist sex worker today; this was her, but back in an age where she could be legitimately stoned to death for her actions. The Bible doesn't explain how she came to be in this profession. There's no knowing whether she made the choice to live way, or if poverty or slavery forced her hand. Either way, her story in Joshua 2:1-24 tells of how she, an outsider and sex worker, turned to Yahweh for help, and He blessed her. Despite her sexual history, despite being of pagan birth and questionable identity, He had mercy on her and saved her life. Not only this, but she also became one of Jesus' ancestors! Don't think God can't use you for His glory just because of your sexual history.

I believe that the Holy Spirit immortalised the accounts of these three people in the Bible for a reason. 1 Timothy 3:16-17 says 'All Scripture is God-breathed and is useful for teaching, rebuking, correcting and training in righteousness …'. I believe these passages are included to remind all humans throughout history that nothing and nobody is irredeemable, that no act is too dirty, sinful or abhorrent to God to lose your forgiveness and salvation.

In fact, some of the figures mentioned earlier were central to God's greatest accomplishment: the birth of Jesus. Both David and Rahab were chosen to be Jesus' ancestors, despite their experiences of sexual sin.

I believe forgiveness is a guarantee and a gift to all who willingly confess their sins and ask for it. It is a sign of the deep, everlasting, reckless, overpowering love of God. The Bible isn't a fairy tale about good people. It's a messy account of a history laden with screw ups, mistakes, sinners and a lot of sexual misconduct! Jesus said He came for the sick, not the healthy.

So why are you excluding yourself from His fantastic grace? He came for you, sister. Just as He shows forgiveness and love to Hosea's wife, King David and Rahab, He wants to forgive you. The only thing holding Him back is you withdrawing from His loving arms in fear.

The beauty of grace is that no one on Earth is worthy of forgiveness. No one lives up to the perfect standard of Yahweh. Only Jesus did this, and yet He was the one who died and sacrificed Himself in order to pay out all of humanities sins. It doesn't make sense, it's not fair. But God chose to perform this great act of kindness and salvation because He loves His created humans so dearly. It isn't something that can be earned, or needs to be worked for, because it's already achieved in the death of Jesus. Relinquish your fear, and know you can be forgiven completely for everything. You are so loved.

3. God is distant, angry and wants to punish me.

This view of God is destructive to your healing. It's impossible to restore intimacy with a figure who you perceive to be angry, dangerous and eager to punish you. The idea that the all-powerful ruler of the universe personally dislikes you is pretty damn depressing … and scary.

If you had a family member or partner hell-bent on punishing you, treating you with contempt and anger, the wise course of action would be to instil boundaries to protect yourself. Perhaps you've done this with God. You can't escape His omniscience and omnipresence, but you may have created unconscious boundaries by removing yourself from Christian community, avoiding prayer or Bible reading and cutting yourself off from the comfort and guidance of God. Some women respond to this perception of God by working hard, too. They focus on 'being good', 'staying out of His way' and slaving over ministry commitments to appease this foreboding God and avoid retribution for their sins.

I wonder where you learned this view of God. Did you have a father figure who was abusive, aloof or demanding? Were you straight out taught that God was distant, angry and punishing? Was fear of God and punishment used against you as spiritual abuse to make you obedient to humans? Did you experience clerical abuse? Or perhaps you need to ask yourself if your own sense of unworthiness is distorting your view of God. Do you feel so unworthy of love and kindness that you've cut yourself off from God? Have you transposed your own assumptions about your self-worth onto Him? Do you believe that someone inherently good and righteous like Jesus could only ever treat you harshly?

If any of these experiences resound with you, I'm so sorry you've been treated with such malice, that you've had to learn to live with this and interpret the world around you through a lens of pain and self-protection.

People can be dangerous, and our own minds can be risky places. I'd like to offer an alternative source for our understanding of God and how He relates to women in pain. It's the same book that David, Gomer and Rahab feature in: the Bible.

I know it's hard to feel connected to an old, religious book a lot of the time. But today, we have the help of the Holy Spirit as well as loads of academic and pastoral resources to help us understand ancient context.

Not only does the Bible speak of God as a Good Father (Matt 7:11) but it contains a particularly culture shattering, feminist tale of sex and affair. I think you might relate.

John 8:1-11

As he was speaking, the teachers of religious law and the Pharisees brought a woman who had been caught in the act of adultery. They put her in front of the crowd.

'Teacher,' they said to Jesus, 'this woman was caught in the act of adultery. The law of Moses says to stone her. What do you say?'

They were trying to trap him into saying something they could use against him, but Jesus stooped down and wrote in the dust with his finger. They kept demanding an answer, so he stood up again and said, 'All right, but let the one who has never sinned throw the first stone!' Then he stooped down again and wrote in the dust.

When the accusers heard this, they slipped away one by one, beginning with the oldest, until only Jesus was left in the middle of the crowd with the woman. Then Jesus stood up again and said to the woman, 'Where are your accusers? Didn't even one of them condemn you?'

'No, Lord,' she said.

And Jesus said, 'Neither do I. Go and sin no more.'

This is not a God of cruelty and punishment. Ours is a God, who came face to face with a woman caught out in sexual sin and spoke freedom into her life. This is the most astounding event, for this woman in particular and all women after her. It says she was 'caught in the act of adultery'. It's not specifically said, but I wonder if she was literally caught in the act. I can imagine these religious men dragging her from the bed she lay in, her desperately trying to cover her body and in an absolute panic. In the days of Jesus, adultery was punishable by death; stoning to be exact. This is what these men were ready to do. They were standing over this woman in her most vulnerable and shameful hour, holding heavy stones ready to bludgeon her to death in judgement. (By the way—where's the dude she's sleeping with? Apparently, he gets off scot free!). Can you just imagine what was going through her head? She would have been experiencing the pinnacle of shame, panic, desperation and fear. Not only was she facing actual death, but her last moments would be swimming in the shame of what she'd done and been caught out doing. She must have felt so small and helpless.

Into this terrifying context, comes Jesus—our Jesus—showing mercy and kindness. He doesn't condemn the woman, He doesn't judge or publicly shame her for her sin, but instead saves her life. He sends the men away by appealing to their logic: 'you who has never sinned may throw the first stone'. They all knew their personal sins, and they walked away. Jesus brings equality. Her sexual sin wasn't more heinous than all these men's (who had no doubt lusted in their hearts many times). All sin, and all people, are invited into grace. My favourite part of this story is that Jesus not only saves her life, but He doesn't even utter any off-handed life advice or patronise her. There's no 'I told you so', 'I can't believe you did that', 'you know you're in the wrong, right?', like we may be tempted to do ourselves, or have been told ourselves. He simply says 'Neither do I [condemn you]. Go and sin no more.' Jesus doesn't brush over sin, He still tells her to pursue change, but He doesn't use punishment, fear or manipulation; He uses freedom and kindness.

This event occurred before Jesus' death and resurrection. How much more mercy shall we anticipate for our sexual sins now, on the other side of the cross? Jesus' death was the punishment to end all punishment, the final act of divine violence and He took it all for you.

Let's not forget the kindness of Jesus. It is available to anyone, anywhere. You don't need to be 'good enough' before coming to Him. You don't have to clean yourself up before approaching him. Remember the woman caught in adultery? She certainly didn't tidy herself up before meeting Jesus, she was thrown in front of him, in her darkest state, and she was met with mercy not anger. Waiting to be 'good enough' before approaching Jesus is like waiting for a gunshot wound to heal before seeking out a doctor.

If this section brought up strong emotions within you, I'm glad. That means old wounds are shifting, and distorted beliefs are making themselves known. These feelings indicate you have some stuff to work through. What is coming up for you? Are you seeing where your understanding of God may have gone awry? Check your inventory timeline and see if you can make any further connections with this spiritual information in mind. It may be time to invest in some spiritual mentors, or distance yourself from others who have been damaging. Our experience of other humans informs our beliefs of God; especially when it comes to relationships, sex and trauma. This is the sick, sad nature of sin.

4. I don't know what I believe anymore. I'm hurt and have doubts.

Rachael was sexually abused by a religious leader in her church when she was young. She was scared, confused and devastated. She discovered porn soon after, and used it to numb her pain. She became addicted, isolated and depressed. She relived the trauma, and sometimes she even fantasised she was the perpetrator, she was in control. Rachael kept it all her secret, as she felt dirty and sinful. As she grew into a young adult, she tried to make the church thing work. She tried to be a good Christian, but none of it felt right. She couldn't shake the horror of what had happened to her—in a church. By a man of 'God', who everyone loved. She grew in bitterness and gave more and more time to her doubts. How could a good God let this happen? How could a Christian do this to her? How could porn be so sinful if it was the only thing comforting her? Unlike God?

She began to read widely and connect with people on a similar spiritual journey. She found it difficult to shake some form of belief in God and an afterlife (mostly because she wanted to see her perpetrator eternally punished) but her doubts began to overpower her. She left the Church, and explored alternative religions and spiritualities.

She didn't know what she believed anymore. She was hurt, and she had big doubts.

Trauma of any kind can shatter your world; it can change the way you engage with people and bring doubts and questions into every relationship and belief in your life. Especially with God. When you survive a devastating event, you suddenly have reason to question the goodness of God. If He is all knowing, all loving, and good, why did He let this happen? If He has a plan, why did He plan something so punishing for you?

These are eternal questions, the centre of apologetics and often the final straw that pushes traumatised women over the precipice of the faith crisis they've been hanging onto for so long. I can't answer these questions for you, nor am I going to attempt to 'defend' God—He can do that Himself. But as you suffer, doubt and question, there are some things I want you to know:

1. Spiritual and sexual abuse by Christian leaders is very real and devastatingly common. If you have been abused or manipulated in any way by a church leader, do not submit to the pressure to stay silent and deny your experience. They are not above the law, or God's judgement.
2. It's okay to have spiritual doubts, to question your religious tradition and think critically. It's also okay to leave the Church if it's hindering your healing.
3. Questioning tradition, interpretations of the Bible, Church culture or Christian leaders doesn't mean you are questioning God or abandoning your faith. Even Jesus questioned the religious leaders of His time.
4. Therapy. Therapy. Therapy! It's not the Devil's work, it's a gift from God!
5. Deconstructing your faith isn't necessarily a bad thing. It is an opportunity to grow and remove traditions that may act as walls between you and Jesus. This is a chance to get to know the real Jesus and own your faith as your own. Continue to journey

with God through this, even if you can't journey with a church right now.

6. It can be extremely traumatic and frightening to walk away from long held beliefs or traditions, and many people won't understand. You may be shunned or shamed, patronised or judged, but you may also be met with kindness, understanding and love. Make sure you don't paint all Christians with the same brush. Either way, if you find yourself in this transitional scenario, equip yourself with strong support. It's out there!

Now what? How do I restore my relationship with Jesus?

There's no formula (unfortunately) for healing your relationship with God. Some religious groups may promise this, but when you turn God into a cookie-cutter formula or a sales-pitch it turns into a whacky Christian incantation or something. It becomes another opportunity for you to feel like a failure when it doesn't work.

The Holy Spirit is the healer. He is the one with the power to draw us closer and closer to God, to reveal truth to us, remind us of the words of Jesus and untangle your distorted view of Him. He will work within every woman in radically different ways. He knows what you need. The stories shared in this chapter have been the personal accounts of unique women, yours will probably look different, and that's okay!

Since I am not the Holy Spirit (thank the Lord, I'm way too unpunctual for that job!), I can't give you a set of instructions guaranteed to 'fix' you or provide an infallible view of God to adhere to. Who's to say I'd be right anyway? I'm still on my own journey to knowing

Jesus better. But I can, however, encourage you to reflect on the views outlined in this chapter, to delve into the Scriptures yourself and meet some of the historical figures who also had messy lives and spur you on to restore genuine intimacy with Jesus. This conversation will be continued in the next chapter as we discuss how to practically restore intimacy with others—including God. I hope you can find what works for your unique relationship with God and wait on Him to pull you into His arms and change your world.

Conclusion

For the woman who feels lonely, drained, forgotten, unworthy, trapped in dead religion and shoulds and should nots—these words are for you. For the woman who is carrying burdens that break your back and your heart, listen. There is an abundance of love for you. There is a God who saw every moment of your life before you were a thought in the universe ... and He still chose to create you, to give you life and be in relationship with you. He saw all of your mess, and still said 'I love her so dearly, my girl!'. He sings over you like a father, and He always has and will never stop. There is safety in His arms, He is unlike any father you've ever known. He wants you to throw off your burdens, your fears and run to Him like a little girl running to her daddy. He doesn't hold condemnation for you, but wants to share intimacy. He wants to hold your hand and walk with you through your recovery and beyond. He has a plan for you—if you'll put down your guard and let Him in. There is nothing you could do to deter God, and there's nothing that needs to be 'fixed' before coming to Him. Right now, in this moment you can lean into His grace and receive His blessings in full.

This is where restoration begins. When the rotten timber is removed from your frame, you can lay a strong foundation upon truth and love. As you continue to read, you will build upon this by increasing intimacy with community and yourself and this will pave the path to your healing. To your restoration.

Action Steps:

1. **Spend some time in prayer. Ask God for clarity and spiritual healing. If this feels too scary right now, simply shoot up a quick request for truth and help or ask a friend to pray for you. He's listening.**
2. **If you haven't yet answered the questions under the heading 'Start at the beginning', do so now. Write them down and reflect on your response.**
3. **Head to The Grace Spot on Spotify and listen to the 'Healing Music' playlist.**

CHAPTER NINE: RESTORING INTIMACY

Restoration. What do you think of when you see that word? When I asked my father-in-law this question, he immediately thought of an old car. He even suggested I use a picture of a broken-down car on the front cover of this book. It took me a while to convince him that may not speak to my target audience! To him, restoration brought up memories of fixing something broken or damaged. He's right—this process involves the hard work and intentionality of 'fixing' what is broken.

However, I personally like to think more in terms of nature. To me, the idea of restoration goes beyond something being 'fixed' and made beautiful again. A car goes from damaged to polished with some elbow grease and love. And it remains that way, its potential is capped. A flowering plant or a powerful tree on the other hand, has unstoppable potential. No matter the storms they weather, the harm inflicted upon their parts, they have the power to regenerate. They're not broken, or damaged goods. They just need a little nurturing to flourish again. And when they do find themselves in an environment conducive to growth, that's exactly what they do. When a plant is restored to life and blooms, they lift their face and stand taller than before. They spread their branches and create a bigger and more beautiful garden for others. Plants that have been pruned back, or knocked about by the wind have the potential to grow beyond what you ever imagined. As they majestically intertwine with the trees around them, they create a newness a stagnant vehicle body will never know. You, my friend, are a precious, budding plant in the world. You may have been roughed up by life, you may feel droopy and broken, but you can be restored. You can flourish and fulfil your full potential, as you were created to do.

Healing from pornography addiction is just as much about adding to your life as it is restricting and eliminating behaviours. Boundaries and rules can keep you sober for a time, but real healing comes when you begin to change your life for the better. You want to create a beautiful life for yourself, one where you have intimate connections with many good people, where you experience genuine joy and satisfaction. Restoration is about creating a life you no longer wish to escape. Intimacy is an essential element to a healthy and whole lifestyle; it is mostly non-sexual and brings the deepest joy and satisfaction.

There are three areas in which a woman recovering from compulsive pornography and chronic shame needs to restore intimacy:

1. With yourself
2. With God
3. With other women and men

I can hear a lot of internal screaming going on. Is that you? The idea of restoring intimacy can be plain frightening—especially if you've experienced trauma.

Stop. Breathe in. Breathe out. Keep breathing.

There's no rush here, and anyway, this isn't a head-first dive into the deep end. In fact, you've probably already started this process of restoration without even knowing it! You've already begun to dip your toes into the icy waters of intimacy, you've just got to keep on edging your feet out deeper and deeper at your own pace.

What do I mean in saying you've already begun?

Well, the practice of restoring intimacy and joy hasn't just been waiting here for you on this page. Way back in the beginning, when you took on an accountability partner and resolved to be honest with yourself and someone else, you were starting to create a new life.

By seeking out accountability you were restoring that intimacy you crave so deeply, but which got lost in the world of porn. You may have also taken my advice to seek a professional therapist or counsellor. Although you pay a professional for their time, this is still a significant relationship in your life and develops your ability to connect. Has it gotten easier in the weeks or months since you took that first step? I hope it has. Intimacy will always involve vulnerability, and by nature that's not easy but I hope it's starting to feel more natural.

Your self-care practices have also been laying a foundation in restoring intimacy and recovering joy. As you've been learning how to rest, be gentle on yourself, practice mindfulness and inner healing you've been getting in touch with the most important person (you! … Okay, second most important if you're a Christian.). When you're deep into porn addiction, you can lose your sense of self-worth and the ability to compassionately connect with yourself and your needs. You've been working on that! Or you've at least read about it and that idea is floating around in your head, which is still great.

This is nothing new for you. But, as we take this topic on head-first, I can't promise you won't hit roadblocks, bumps and potholes. I certainly did! These will be different for every woman. Some may have to deal with the effects of assault while they attempt to reconnect with their world, others may be dealing with the complexities of their sexuality, mental illness, cultural barriers or unsafe family environments. Most women struggling with pornography will have some kind of relational wounding which will need to be dealt with as they work on restoring intimacy.

However, we all need to replace darkness with joy and life, and there are common practices, fears and questions that arise when committing to this process. These will be outlined in the coming chapter and come from my own experiences and those of other women who have graciously shared with me.

1. Restoring intimacy with yourself

Intimacy with yourself isn't as dirty as it sounds. This is less about pleasuring yourself and more about caring for yourself. Restoring intimacy with yourself involves reclaiming your identity, acknowledging your feelings and attending to your basic emotional and physical needs (self-care!). It's about feeling at home within yourself.

Restoring intimacy by: Reclaiming your identity

The shame that lives in the shadow of pornography has a way of eating away at your identity. It spits poisonous lies about your worth and convinces you to forget who you really are. Instead of a multi-faceted, valuable human being with important needs and aspirations, you identify as a 'worthless porn addict' or something similarly self-deprecating. Shame convinces us we are worthless; we are bad people and nothing more. You lose your sense of self and your identity becomes skewed.

Part of restoring intimacy with yourself is getting to know yourself again. Akin to restoring intimacy with a friend or lover, you must invest time, understanding, vulnerability and unconditional love into this journey. You can reclaim your identity from the grips of porn and shame by giving time to exploring your personality. This is about discovering who you are outside of being a porn user, or someone experiencing pain. There is much, much more to you than your struggle.

You can work on this by writing a physical list or mind-map of your interests, talents and unique character traits. Ask your friends or family, whoever knows you best, to give their input too. What makes you special to them? They often see what's in our personal blind spots. Don't forget to acknowledge God through this as well, and seek spiritual guidance (from a friend, mentor or pastor). Who does God say you are? What does He say about you? How can you live out your God-given identity?

Restoring intimacy by: Acknowledging feelings and emotions

If you were spending time with a friend, and constantly ignoring or stifling their emotions and feelings, you wouldn't be a very good friend, would you? You wouldn't truly get to know them, because you would be avoiding intimacy and vulnerability. Consider it the same when it comes to restoring intimacy with yourself. Be kind to yourself by letting yourself feel what you feel without judgment or repression. It can feel overwhelming, but every time you practice this you become more at home with yourself. By shutting down emotions and feelings you create distance within yourself. We discussed this kind of mindfulness in chapter seven, if you'd like to revisit it now.

Hopefully you've already been doing the groundwork for this practice as you've been reading about it. If you've been neglecting self-care and mindfulness, now is the time to revisit those previous chapters and give it a go.

Restoring intimacy by: Attending to physical & emotional needs

Intimacy means being fully known and fully loved. By reclaiming your identity and acknowledging your emotional needs, you're half-way to restoring intimacy with yourself. The second part of this process is about treating yourself with the unconditional love and respect you desire from an outside source. It's about prioritising self-care, even if you feel like you don't deserve it. Self-care was outlined in detail in chapter three.

We're starting with the self as it's probably the least steep slope to slide down into this new world of healthy connections. It's by no means a simple task for a recovering porn addict who's used to escaping reality rather than engaging with her needs, but it only involves you. We're starting small and building up to connecting with the world again.

2. Restoring intimacy with God

The previous chapter tackled distorted views of God and made an attempt to distinguish between nasty legalism or religion and the gracious kindness of Jesus. We identified spiritual abuse, too, which can have devastating effects on the life and faith of women. It was a call to reassess your spiritual state and why you may hold certain beliefs about yourself, God or the Church. I provided some possible alternative beliefs to common misconceptions of God—such as He couldn't love me, He's angry or distant or maybe isn't even there at all. I do hope thinking through some of those spiritual barriers has made you feel confident enough to start moving closer to Jesus and restoring intimacy with Him.

This spiritual connection is powerfully healing. When you feel the love, validation, acceptance and forgiveness of the one who created every speck of dust in the universe, it's pretty special. This is the truest form of intimacy, because God is the only one who truly and fully knows you. There are no secrets, no hidden things to Him. Every image you've seen, every thought, action and desire is plain to him. He knows the number of hairs on your head (He even knows how much of it falls out into the bathroom sink every week) and every strand of DNA is familiar to Him. To be known that intimately is life-changing.

But how on earth do you experience this? So many of us grew up chanting Sunday school songs like 'Jesus loves me this I know, for the Bible tells me so …' and every women's conference smacks you in the face with floral Bible verses telling of your worth and value. I mean, the whole 'Jesus loves you' vibe is so common it's even printed on bouncy balls at the local Christian book shop. We know it in our heads, but sometimes it feels impossible to truly believe.

Each woman's walk with Jesus is unique and I can't snap my fingers and make you feel genuinely loved, valued and known by the Divine. If I could, my fingers would be blistered to the bone from snapping all day, every day, for my beautiful sisters.

But God will take you on a restorative journey if you ask Him. It may take years—scratch that—it *will* take years. Our sanctification is an ongoing and ever-changing process. The spiritual walk is wrought with ups, downs, twists and turns and just when you think you've got it all together—or lost it all—God will whoosh you into another world and show you so much more than you ever imagined. He's got you girl. He's holding your hand and cheering you on as you pursue Him more and more!

I entered into a healing intimacy with God over many years which began through a long conversation with a Christian friend on a road trip, a poignant song and a single, red tulip. Charli's walls were broken down through childbirth and parenting; Evie had a powerful dream where she spoke with Jesus and it changed everything in her waking life; Brodie came to find peace and closeness with the God of her childhood through therapy and talking through her spiritual roadblocks. We are all so different, and have different needs. God knows this and is the instigator of all healing.

While you can't manipulate God or force His hand to heal and restore you—or even improve your relationship with Him—you *can* ask Him. In fact, sometimes you won't even need to ask; in all of the previous cases, it was totally unexpected for the women in question.

There are also several other practices which may further put you in a place of spiritual wellness, openness and connection with God.

The following list isn't exhaustive, and none of these practices are necessarily required to connect with God and experience intimacy, but they can definitely help.

- Read the Bible (Classic Christian solution amiright?).
- Spend time in prayer. Talk to God and listen for Him in the peace and quiet.
- Journal, draw or paint your prayers and spiritual thoughts (even if they're dark).
- When you pray, imagine Jesus is sitting in front of you, rather than hiding in the ceiling somewhere. Talk to Him like a friend or mentor, not a cloud in the sky.

- Listen to worship music. Let it wash over you. Sing and dance if you want.
- Flee from people and practices that turn God into a dead, legalistic religion of shame.
- Focus more on Jesus than rules, guilt and 'good behaviour'.
- Don't be afraid to explore books or podcasts that question the religion or tradition of your upbringing. Trust the Holy Spirit to guide you to truth.
- Disconnect from distractions for a while. Put away the technology, and allow yourself space to be alone with your thoughts and God
- Connect with a Christian community that is genuinely loving and allows you to be free.
- Allow yourself to be vulnerable with other Christians about your spiritual, emotional and physical struggles. Give others permission to do the same; God can teach you a lot through honest conversations with others.

I know some of these recommendations have probably been used to guilt you in the past. Some of them are classically oversimplified Christian solutions to very real and complex issues, and they may have made you cringe. Like, really? Reading my Bible is going to fix my porn problem and my spiritual trauma? Ha!

I know some of these practices are the last thing you feel like doing when you're disconnected and dubious about God, and I know that none of them guarantee you'll feel better at all. My intention is not to guilt you, or oversimplify the complexities of a spiritual physical existence, but to remind you that these suggestions are here, and they all can help you reconnect with God (mostly through the Holy Spirit, rather than by the practice itself). They're also certainly not isolated practices. Holistic healing for a woman struggling with porn encapsulates everything in the previous eight chapters, including therapy and trauma work if needed. Restoring intimacy with God is an important aspect to healing, but it's not the entire picture and will look unique for every woman.

Find what works for you; a relationship with Jesus is as unique as any other relationship between two people. It's not something you can prescribe through a set of rules or recommendations. And remember, never shame yourself into 'good Christian behaviour' simply because you feel you must keep up a good image: that's not intimacy, that's religion.

3. Restoring intimacy with other people

If this restoring thing was a game, you've reached Level Ten. We're on hard-mode now. We're going to restore intimacy with other people.

This is much easier said than done. This is often the most frightening part of the process, because it involves actual vulnerability with other people. Reconnecting with men and women carries inherent risk. Humans are capable of inflicting pain and increasing shame. We can't control other people's actions. You may have first-hand knowledge of that. For women who have been abused, mistreated or otherwise traumatised at the hands of another human, the idea of breaking out of that safe little cocoon of isolation and presenting yourself to the world again can be daunting. Everything in your body and mind tells you to hide and never ever put yourself at risk of being hurt again.

Tash knows the difficulty in reconnecting.

I was terrified of humiliation and to me, that experience was always just around the corner. I didn't know how to engage with people, especially men. My only experience with them had ended in pain and embarrassment. So I hid, I cried and made excuses not to attend events where I'd feel uncomfortable ... even though I so desperately sought love, community and friendship. The thing I wanted most was the thing that terrified me and sent my anxiety into a frenzy. I would often end up going back to pornography to comfort this pain and fantasise about being close to another person.

There's no shame in this struggle. Your anxiety is proof that your brain and body are working as they should. When you touch a hot frying pan, your brain sends signals to your body to recoil and avoid experiencing that pain again. After being burnt, you'll develop a healthy hesitation around hot cooking equipment. Your brain does the same thing when it comes to emotional pain and trauma. It's trying to protect you.

The problem is, a hot frying pan will always be dangerous; intimacy with another person isn't. Connection is actually the thing that can heal our wounds. Our brain finds it difficult to distinguish between safe and unsafe people though, so in order to protect, it tends to stay on high alert around everyone.

Restoring intimacy is quite a challenge, as it involves pushing back on our neurological signals. It does get easier with practice. As your brain starts to associate social interaction and vulnerability with positive benefits, it will calm down. At the beginning, it may feel like you're fighting against yourself. Working with a psychologist can be a huge help at this stage, too. Your therapist and accountability partner are a great sounding board to debrief about your experiences, as well as being available to help you determine appropriate boundaries and identify safe places and people to connect with. Developing strong and wise boundaries is a vital skill a recovering woman must learn.

So where should you start? There's no need to jump straight in the deep end; start with the people you already know. Develop your existing friendships or focus on deepening your connection with an acquaintance who could turn into a good friend. If you have safe family members, invest in quality time with them, too. After you practice this for a while, you can move on to more challenging tasks, like meeting new people.

Write down your existing friendships or others you have some kind of connection with. Who can you start reconnecting with?

When it comes to meeting new people, it's important to be wise and set boundaries. You know your personal triggers, so identify those and avoid them. It may be alcohol, drugs, shirtless men, certain language, music or the late night that inhibits your recovery. You might need to ask your friends not to discuss certain things around you, or choose to stay in, rather than hit the clubs. Keeping this in mind, when you feel ready to venture a little further out into recovery-land and make some more healing connections, there are three groups of people who will be beneficial to your recovery: female friends, support groups and your family of choice.

Female friendships

Female friendships are an important aspect of recovery for women. These relationships provide a wonderful, safe place to practice vulnerability and re-learn trust in a platonic way free from the messiness of romance and sexual tension. It is important to restore friendships with men eventually; this is the only way you will learn how to relate healthily towards the opposite gender. But for now, focusing on female friendships can be less triggering and frightening than engaging with unfamiliar men. Your gal pals will also become an invaluable source of support when you do venture into the world of male friendships and dating. Build up a strong foundation with them first, unless you have strong existing male friendships which support your healing.

For women who identify as LGBTQI+, it may be a little different. As a cis-gendered, heterosexual woman, I am not an expert on recovery for LGBTQI+ people, but the advice regarding accountability for same-sex attracted women could well be applied here. Female friendships remain vital for recovery, but focus on developing platonic friendships with women you aren't romantically interested in, to avoid complication as you heal.

There are some difficulties involved in engaging with other women that you should be aware of. Porn actresses are usually portrayed as overtly sexualised and submissive; porn-land is not a place of equality and respect. Women only exist for pleasure. This can lead to confusing and unwanted sexualisation or attraction towards female friends in otherwise heterosexual women. It can also lead to shame for 'letting down the sisterhood' by your participation in their exploitation. Further complications arise when you find yourself relating far more with your friend's male partner who struggles with pornography, than her. In moments like these, your femininity may feel compromised and conversation could become awkward or shaming. It's not easy connecting back into your old friendship circle, or forging your way in a new one, but it's worth it. The prevailing rumour about women is that they are bitchy and backstabbers, that they don't make good friends. But I think you'll find that most women are just seeking a friend to share life with. We all feel alone in this world and most women are more than eager to join forces with one another and share the love. Engage with healthy and safe female social circles and be patient with yourself as you 'reprogram' your mind.

The further you get away from porn—and the closer to genuine friendships—the easier it will become to live free and embrace restoration.

Support groups

Support groups are a fantastic tool for women wanting to restore real relationships. Not only do they provide accountability, understanding, a structured program and encouragement for overcoming porn, they are a huge source of safe, healthy intimacy. There's not much more healing than sitting in a (digital or real) room of women who have walked the same walk you have. It can be nerve-racking to begin with, but the shared experience creates a safety unlike anything else and provides a place where women are comfortable to share their deepest secrets, regrets and hopes for the future. These groups are places where deep and lasting intimacy can be practiced. It becomes a sisterhood, a family. These are women who become lifelong friends and who understand you better than you may even understand yourself at times. Joining a support group is a sure-fire way to practice and rebuild intimacy in a safe environment. Groups can be found online, in person and by phone call in some places. Some groups are listed on The Grace Spot under 'Get Help' followed by 'Get Accountable'. To find local groups, a quick internet search including your location should suffice.

Jenny says this about restoring intimacy in a support group setting:

It's [connecting with others] something I still really struggle with. One thing that has helped is learning to set boundaries. That makes me feel a little safer in trying to develop friendships. The other thing that has been helpful is attending a women's twelve-step group. Going out for breakfast after the meeting and occasionally doing a social activity with the women gives me a chance to practice social interaction with others in a safe way.

Family of choice

Another important way to reconnect is through what Marnie Ferree calls your 'family of choice'[1 (p.193)]. If your own parents did not and cannot fulfil your needs for comfort, love, safety and intimacy, look for a family you can 'join'. It doesn't matter how old you are, a supportive family is key to healing, even if they're not related by blood. This is one of the best aspects of being part of a church community. Part of the Christian mandate is to care for widows, orphans and the needy. This includes emotional orphans, too! You'll find there are many older couples and families eager to adopt single women, mentor outcasts and embrace those who need a loving set of parents or grandparents. You may also find your family of choice outside of the Christian community—through family friends, community programs or work. You may even have a close female friend whose family takes you in as their own daughter.

Emily, a thirty-three-year-old woman, connected on a deep level with her Bible study leaders, an older married couple with two teenage children. They made time to invite Emily over for meals, take her on outings and even financially support her when she was in dire need. They knew her history and understood she had a parent-shaped hole in her heart. Emily became part of the family, and at her wedding her 'Bible study Dad' even walked her down the aisle. This family was the safest and most loving place she ever knew, and it, along with regular therapy was foundational in her healing from pornography addiction and childhood trauma.

Small steps

For many women, intentionally socialising and inviting intimacy into their lives is overwhelming. It's scary and it can be hard to know where to start. Talk this over with a professional counsellor, your mentor or accountability partner and know your journey will be unique. But here are a few tips to encourage you to just start reconnecting:

- Take small steps. Start by working within your current friendships. Choose one friend to focus on at a time. How can you connect with them this week or month?
- It doesn't have to be a big event, or highly organised. Simply invite a friend or two out for coffee and cake.
- Reconnecting can begin with a simple text or online message saying 'Hey! How are you?'.
- You should already have an accountability partner or small group. Think of ways you can develop these friendships and encourage them.
- Allow yourself to attend events and leave early without guilt. If you're anxious, tell yourself you can just go for one hour and come home—and that's okay!

- If you're anxious about larger events or gatherings, bring along your closest friend and tell them you're unsettled. Ask for moral support.
- Think of a hobby or activity you once loved and give it a second chance.
- Or, take a friend along to something totally new!
- How is your relationship with church community? Can you invest in these friendships by joining a small group or staying after the sermon for a little longer to chat?
- Be kind to yourself and celebrate every tiny victory. What you're doing is brave.
- Try just saying 'yes' to an event invitation and see what happens. You might just have the time of your life.
- Is there an online support group you can join with other women?
- Smile at strangers as you walk by each other, even say hello or good morning/afternoon if you're feeling brave!
- Ask a stranger for directions or recommendations for the best coffee in the area instead of heading straight for Google.
- Head for the check-out with a real human manning it, rather than self-serve if you've got emotional energy.

Can you think of any more ways you can gently reengage with the world? Write them down and set yourself some challenges!

Dating, marriage and sex

Self-care, God-time and friendships are all well and good, but what about … *intimacy intimacy*? What happens when a recovering porn addict wants to take the next step and dive into dating? What about when the time comes for marriage and sex? Will their sexual history ruin the wedding night? Should they tell their partner all those dirty little secrets on the first date? These are common questions from recovering women who have their eyes set on the future, and they need to be addressed.

My advice to unmarried women who want to know if they'll ever have a good marriage with good sex is to slow down. My friend, it's amazing to hear you're feeling so free and so ready to start thinking about the future, but you're not there yet (unless you're currently engaged—then we can talk sex!). For now, focus on your recovery. Focus on healing, reflecting on your personal pain and building up strong friendships with women and men. Give yourself all the time you need to truly heal and flourish, don't rush the romance. You may end up doing more harm to yourself than good, and be mindful that your marriage anxiety could be another expression of your false core beliefs. Do you remember false belief number three? Sex is a necessity to feel good. It's great to hope for a healthy and fulfilling marriage one day, but if you are pinning all your recovery hopes and dreams on having sex, you might be going astray in your healing. Check in with yourself about if you need to push back on that belief, and if you genuinely believe you can have a whole, restored and happy life if you never get married or have sex. Maybe that's the issue you need to work on right now, rather than trying to sort out your future sex life.

From my experience, I can say the best marriages come from a deep and organic friendship. I was a chronic crusher in my day, always obsessed with some guy I just met and planning our future wedding on Pinterest. I was constantly on high alert for that future hubby I had been praying for to fix me and my loneliness. I tried to force it to happen so many times, and it only left me feeling awkward and hurt. As it turns out, God was protecting me from all my crushes. He had the perfect guy already waiting for me. Lukas had been one of my closest friends for over seven years before we started dating. He wasn't on my romantic radar at all until the timing was right—eight years after we had initially met. Our long and genuine friendship has been the foundation for a wonderful, intimate marriage and it has helped us improve our sex life with humour, patience and love. Focus on friendships and recovery right now, and let romance happen in time. I am still constantly reminding myself is to stay in the season I am currently in. Whether it's singleness, dating, engagement, marriage, starting a family or the next career move, we always seem to be looking ahead and, as a result, miss out on enjoying our current stage of life. I call it 'season jumping' and it robs women of joy and contentment. Be free to dream of the future, but don't try to force change or deal with theoretical future issues before they even arise. Fully embrace the season you're in, especially when it comes to recovery.

I know some of you still just want me to answer the damn question, and offer some advice, so I will. But you may not like my response. I'm not giving you a straight yes or no, but I'm going to let you in on a little marriage secret instead …

The question 'will porn/a sexual history ruin my wedding night?' is totally flawed, because it's based on the premise that wedding-night sex is supposed to be perfect, that it's something that can be 'ruined' by one minor mishap. The intense fear that exists around the thought of 'messing up' your wedding night really reveals just how much expectation is placed on that one experience. It's as if glorious newly-wed sex is some kind of promise or reward for waiting, for recovering, for being a good Christian girl. I wonder where that idea came from? (*Cough, purity culture, cough*).

Porn addiction or a sexual history can only ruin your honeymoon if you let it. It can only destroy your first encounter with married sex if your expectations are for perfection. These expectations are the thing that's really going to ruin your wedding night.

Christianity needs to re-evaluate what it's teaching young people. Wedding-night sex (and honeymoon sex, and the first year of sex in general) isn't great. It's not perfection. Sure, it's special, but it's likely not going to be the best sex of your life. It's probably going to be a little awkward, confusing and difficult. It involves learning an entirely new skill and coordinating together with another person who is also learning, and possibly anxious. A lot of young married couples don't even experience an orgasm for a few months after tying the knot—it's an art, and although it may be easy enough for you to experience one on your own, learning how to do that for and with another person takes effort and patience. Honestly, this mutual struggle is the real beauty of sex. Great intercourse isn't about having a perfect physical experience, but is about sharing intimacy and learning together. There is so much vulnerability involved in working through your struggles in marriage—whether they're related to porn, masturbation and previous experiences or something entirely different. Everyone brings baggage to the marriage bed, not just women struggling with pornography. This shared vulnerability is what makes sex special, not having perfect orgasms. If you're willing to learn together, communicate with your spouse and be honest about your struggles, you can't ruin your wedding night or future sex life.

This isn't to say you won't need or shouldn't utilise support for your specific issues. On the contrary, If needed, I enthusiastically encourage women to access sex therapy, couples counselling and use resources created for specific issues such as trauma, anxiety, vaginismus, PTSD, arousal issues and many more. There's no shame in seeking outside support to help you and your marriage thrive!

The F word

It's time to discuss the F word! No, not that one. We're moving on from that. If you need more sex and marriage advice, head to The Grace Spot for resources, but now we're going to talk about FUN! Good, clean fun! Pursuing fun, frivolity and joy is part of recovery, and can make all the difference in your healing.

Fun is underrated. When was the last time you remember having fun? How often do you see 'little fun'—making light of a situation, laughing, random bites of surprise and joy—in your daily life? What about 'bigger fun'? When was the last time you went on a holiday? Had an adventure? Belly laughed with a friend or squealed with surprise? What gives you life and how can you do more of it? Fun can be a wonderful antidote to fear, stress, anger, depression and isolation. Therapy, accountability, medication and recovery work are necessary processes too, don't hear me wrong. But a belly laugh is medicine that can never be prescribed too much. Joy is a healing thing, it takes you out of the dark places in your mind and can make you forget your troubles, even if just for a little while.

This is where reengaging or starting new group hobbies can be of huge benefit to your recovery. Is there a regular, fun, community activity you can join in on? These have all the benefit of fun and help you engage with new relationships. It could be baking, gardening, writing, art, restoring old cars, dancing, camping or cleaning. It could be anything that brings you joy! I am a huge advocate in particular for women picking up some form of health or fitness hobby during recovery. Joining a gym, walking club, training for a marathon, taking up yoga, unicycling, swimming, powerlifting or any number of other physical activities give you a triple prize: improved physical wellbeing, fun and human connection. All of these things make you feel great, and when you feel great, you have so much less reason to turn to porn. Another reason why I love fitness related activities is their ability to encourage women to take up space and set and achieve practical goals. This can give you a great boost of self-confidence and bolster your porn recovery. If you can work up to lifting 100kg weights or running 42 kilometres, you can keep fighting porn! I found this to be integral to my own healing. I joined a roller derby team and took up powerlifting as a way to reengage with the world and avoid isolation. It was terrifying at first, but the communities that surround both these sports embraced me, became my personal cheer squad, and friends. They made me feel worthwhile, unlike anything else I had ever done. Trust me, when you're attempting a heavy lift for the first time or win a roller derby match and your teammates are cheering your name, it's incredibly validating and healing. You are known, you are loved, you are supported, you are strong!

Maybe it's the same in a maths or puzzle club, but I wouldn't know.

Whatever fun means to you, pursue it. It's part of healing.

Conclusion

When you risk rejection by opening yourself up to intimacy—through friendships, with God, through support groups, families of choice, community activities and even with yourself—you can effectively challenge your core beliefs (remember them? Your tree roots!). When you receive enough acceptance and love, and develop strong friendships, you forge new self-beliefs that focus on positivity, value and hope. When you experience grace and forgiveness from human hands, it becomes easier to trust in God's grace and forgiveness for you. Restoring intimacy is the final piece of the puzzle. It has the power to draw together all you've learned so far, and all the hard work you've done, and tie it together in a neat and restorative bow.

Can you see hope shimmering through the darkness? (Maybe with a bit of fear too—that's okay). I hope so. I want you to see there is hope. You can have a beautiful future. No matter what age or stage you're at right now, despite your addiction and all the pain you feel, you can flourish and bloom. You can have deep and satisfying relationships, and engage with the world without shame holding you back! You can experience the power of love and acceptance, by both others, God and yourself. Right now, you may feel isolated, lonely and unworthy of love and connection. I've been there. Many women have. In fact, underneath all the smiles and expensive eye-makeup, most women out there probably feel this rumbling in their hearts, too. So, let's join together and love on one another. Let's reach out, accept others, speak life and put ourselves out there in vulnerability. Let's restore intimacy in our lives, and eradicate the need for faux intimacy on screen. Let's challenge our, and each other's, core beliefs and restore words of wisdom, love and gratitude to our hearts. You deserve to take up space in this world and make a difference with your unique abilities and capability for love. There is so much out there in the world for you to experience, and I know you have the courage within you to take that first step and reach out.

Action Steps:

1. **Reflect on your unique characteristics. What makes you, you? Express this creatively through art, journaling, mind mapping or a simple list.**
2. **List your existing friendships to help you identify who you can intentionally reconnect with easily. For more of a challenge, write down where you might be able to meet new friends.**
3. **If your family are unavailable in any way, write down some options for a 'family of choice'.**
4. **Write a list of hobbies and interests that appeal to you or you used to participate in. Make a plan to re-engage with these.**

CHAPTER TEN: OVERCOMING SHAME

Did you skip ahead to this chapter?
It's alright if you did, I expected some women to! Shame is a woman's arch nemesis. More than the compulsive porn use itself or any other behaviours, shame is the feeling that overwhelms a porn user. Every woman I've ever met who struggled with porn or masturbation to any degree has emphasised the feelings of shame that shackle her to silence and addiction. Of course a chapter titled 'Overcoming Shame' is going to jump right out and scream 'turn to me!'. Unfortunately, if you've dropped yourself right into chapter ten without any prior reading, this isn't going to work for you. Sorry to burst your bubble, but there's no magic remedy, no secret incantation, no special potion or prayer that can immediately take away your deep feelings of shame.

But there is hope.

That hope comes in the form of a process, a journey, and it culminates with sharing your own story with the world and serving others.

If you attempt this without any prior recovery work, you're probably going to have a bad time. It takes both resilience and a basic understanding of where we've been throughout this recovery guide to tackle shame effectively. So, if you've come here first, this is your 'WRONG WAY, GO BACK' sign. At least for the time being. Head back to chapter one and settle in the for the journey.

If that spiel was irrelevant for you and you're up to chapter ten of this journey, welcome! You've been doing the hard work of digesting all this information, and hopefully putting some of it into practice—that's no small feat. Now you're ready to discuss what it looks like to overcome shame.

What is shame?

I bet I don't need to describe what shame feels like for you to know it. I'm sure it's a constant companion on your shoulder, a familiar but heavy burden that feels like poison in your veins. It inhibits your vision for a future, for hope, for freedom. It convinces you to hide, stay silent and lock your doors to the world, it whispers degrading things in your ear and constantly reminds you of every negative thing that's ever been said or done to you. It reminds you to stay small and continue in your addiction. Shame researcher and author Brené Brown, describes shame as 'the intensely painful feeling or experience of believing we are flawed and therefore unworthy of love and belonging.'[1]

For me, shame manifested in many ways, but often it was a snide, nasty voice inside my head. It would say:

'You're disgusting.'

'You're useless.'

'Everyone is laughing at you.'

'You look stupid.'

'You deserve pain.'

What does shame say to you?

Do you remember the addiction tree from chapter six? Shame can be found in every part of it, but most clearly in the roots. The roots represented the four core beliefs of a female addict:

1. I am a bad person, unworthy of love
2. No one will ever love me as I am
3. Sex is a necessity to feel good
4. My needs will never be met by anyone else

Those are the voices of shame.

They were our simplest way of understanding our unique traumas, abandonments and pain. Often, these stem from childhood and become swollen with age. The longer you believe these things, the truer they seem. More events occur that seem to confirm these beliefs, and addiction is the final straw that solidifies the shame. We've learned, however, that those beliefs are faulty. They are coping mechanisms for trauma or pain that transcend our ability to cope. These came from the outside, and have only caused damage. This means that with some deconstruction, shame can be overcome.

Okay so how do I do it then?! Where do I start?

Guess what? If you've been actively participating in this recovery guide, you've already begun the journey. At its core, overcoming shame is the challenging of fundamental beliefs about yourself and the world. It's fighting distorted views that say you're worthless and alone. This has been central to every chapter of *Restored*. The starter pistol has fired and you've left the mark. You're running this race already! But recovery is a long-distance event, so don't stop now.

Everything we've discussed thus far can help you overcome shame. By giving time and commitment to the practices outlined in this guide, over time your shame will ebb away. Since much of our shame had its beginnings in childhood or early adolescence, don't expect an instant fix. Expect to work hard. As frustrating as this is, there *is* a silver lining to the complexity of healing. The intentionality required to overcome your insecurities and toxic thinking builds character and wisdom. The process will serve to build you up and make you more assertive, reflective and mindful. You will gain insight not only into your own troubled mind but will develop the ability to recognise pain in others and empower them to heal though the lessons learned in your own journey.

The practices (as outlined in previous chapters) I recommend you focus on and continue returning to in order to overcome shame are as follows:

Continued accountability and therapy

Accountability and therapy were discussed in chapter two. Dr. Brené Brown says 'the less we talk about shame, the more power it has over our lives. If we cultivate enough awareness about shame to name it and speak to it, we've basically cut it off at the knees'[2] (p.53). Getting beyond shame means acknowledging it and sharing your experience with trusted people in your life, such as your accountability partner, therapist or mentor. These are the people who know you aren't perfect but love you anyway. These relationships are wonderful places to practice vulnerability through your ongoing honesty about pornography—which in itself tackles shame—plus, they also provide an open space to share about the impact of shame on your life. Their listening ear and outside input can give you a sense of perspective on your shame and can help you come up with strategies to deal with it. A therapist will have professional practices to support you, while an accountability partner or mentor can provide you with a more intimate kind of support and encouragement as you journey. Remember, shame thrives in secrecy and isolation. Kill it by letting it out into the open.

Mindfulness

Mindfulness was discussed in chapter seven.

When dealing with shame, Thomas Scheff wrote for the *Journal of Cultural Sociology* that 'Shame is the most obstructed and hidden emotion, and therefore the most destructive. Emotions are like breathing—they cause trouble only when obstructed'[3].

Do you remember the concept of noticing and describing your emotions as you would a painting on the wall or a piece of furniture in the house? This is how you can bring shame out of hiding, and prevent it from obstructing healthy function. It must be acknowledged, in order to remove its power.

'That lounge is green and soft; it has two cushions with sequins on them.'

'I feel ashamed that I didn't raise my hand in class to ask the question I wanted to. I felt embarrassed to be seen.'

'I feel like everyone knows how anxious I am. I feel like they think I'm stupid. I feel embarrassed'.

'I fell on the sidewalk in front of a crowd. I feel embarrassed. I feel like everyone is laughing at me.'

By identifying your emotions and feelings before shame descends, you can beat the shame cycle that spirals you out of control into acting out behaviour. If you don't pause, breathe and carefully identify your emotions, you run the risk of shame piling up and, rather than being able to identify what *actually* happened, how you *actually* feel and *why*, shame grabs a speakerphone and screams 'you are worthless, you are crap, you're a fool, everyone is judging you!'. That never helps.

In order to overcome shame, continue practicing mindfulness and reaching out for more resources to assist you in practicing this.

Inner Child work

Many distorted beliefs we hold about ourselves find their origin in childhood. Not always, but often. Our inner child often missed out on safety, nurturing or intimacy. Shame can be a long-known companion. Shame and self-blame are a child's way of understanding pain. A child doesn't have the cognitive ability to understand that bad things can happen because someone else (usually a parent or caregiver) has done something wrong. In their world, the only sensible logic is that they have done something wrong—they are to blame or they are not loved. A young person will seek answers to understand the pain they experience, even if they are damning, rather than living in uncertainty or confusion.

For example, my dad was emotionally and spiritually absent from my life. Physically, he was mostly around. But emotionally, there was a wall between us. I don't have memories of hearing 'I love you' or other shows of affection and validation. I didn't feel known or valued by him. This didn't make sense to me. How could a dad who was physically present feel so absent? Why wasn't he treating me the way I saw other fathers treat their daughters? I had been taught that parents were all-knowing, all-good and all-loving. But this wasn't my experience. In order to realign my understanding of the world with reality I concluded that I, as the child, must be the problem. I must be unlovable—I must be flawed in some way if he couldn't love me as I desired. I carried this belief well into adulthood and it impacted my romantic relationships. It took rigorous counselling and mentoring for me to understand he had actually wronged me, not the other way around. Only with professional outside support was I able to understand the impact chronic pain, medication, mental health and his own upbringing had on my father's ability to parent.

As outlined in chapter seven, nurture your inner child. As a grown woman, be who you needed as a girl. Comfort, nurture, care for and play on behalf of that hurt little girl within. Tell her she is loved and worthy. Acknowledge whatever damage was done to her as a child was wrong. We are all a little girl within a woman's body. Don't forget her. She carries shame that you as a grown woman have the power to speak into.

Restoring intimacy

This was discussed in chapter nine.

This is a 'level up' from accountability and therapy. This is about taking the relational skills you've developed with a support person into the world and restoring intimacy in healthy, safe friendships and communities. Isolation is like fuel thrown on a flame: it feeds shame and causes it to explode. With every friendship you invest into with care, your world widens. You begin to see outside of your own troubles and gain perspective. You see that other people make mistakes too, but you still love them. Over time you should be able to translate these life lessons into self-acceptance.

As you begin to take up more space in the world, as you grow bolder and deeper in relationships, you will gain a new collection of evidence that proves to your brain that you can be safe, loved and intimate without disaster. You're currently functioning off experiences of vulnerability leading to pain and fear, and feeling shame about these. New experiences can help you overcome that shame. Give it time to accumulate, but your brain will slowly begin to see the difference—especially if you're also deconstructing your trauma and experiences with a mentor, accountability partner, recovery resource or therapist.

As you develop friendships and relationships that flourish, you will start to believe what these people are saying to you: that you are worthy of love and affection. That your needs can be met without sex. That you are not rejected or hated, but loved and accepted.

Pursuit of intimacy with God

Another version of my most frequently asked question ('How do I deal with shame?') is 'How do I feel forgiven?'. A woman might be doing great recovery work, have sobriety under her belt and have faith in God, but her inability to accept forgiveness shackles her to shame. This only multiplies as women succumb to the guilt of not being a 'good believing Christian'.

Before getting into how to 'solve' this issue, let me say that it's okay you feel this. It's okay that you experience the inconsistency of being both a Christ-follower and a doubter. It isn't pleasant or ideal, but a little uncertainty is part of being a human who follows a currently invisible God. I guess that's why it's called 'faith'.

Don't let this scare you. In these times of doubt, remember your salvation and ongoing relationship with Jesus hasn't anything to do with you and your behaviour. It is God who does the forgiving and healing, it is He who holds onto you during these times of uncertainty. No one is deserving of His magnificent grace and kindness, and yet He offers it freely to anyone who will come to Him, including you.

If you're still really struggling with this spiritual shame, I encourage you to head back to chapter eight. This chapter dealt with restoring intimacy with God and examining your view of who He is. This can help you reflect on the 'why' behind feelings of shame and not being forgiven, and assist in wiping distorted views of God out of the cobwebbed attic of your mind and reconnecting with the Jesus who came specifically to embrace the sick and lost. This is where healing occurs.

Again, there's no formula here. This is about your personal relationship with God, and how much you allow Him to work on your bruised and battered heart. He wants to gently unravel the wounds within you that shield you from accepting His forgiveness and freedom. He wants to unpick those tight knots within you that grew out of fear and trauma.

Be persistent in pursuing intimacy with God. Allow yourself to be loved in the middle of the mess by meditating through worship music, reading Bible passages that speak to you and spending time listening to God in the silence, rather than with the toxic voices in your head.

Overcoming shame is also about sharing your story

Stories have the power to crack open our hearts so the spirit of God can flow through our innermost being. For the storyteller, and their audience, stories are often an untapped source of powerful change and healing. You don't need to be 'fully healed' or have your life together in order to participate in the healing power of storytelling. Testimonies can be shared at any stage. In fact some of the most meaningful and impactful tales I've heard have been from women who are still 'works-in-progress'. You're not disqualified from using your voice to share if your story doesn't yet have the pretty pink ribbon tying everything together at the end. Messy stories are real and valuable, and they help both you and others heal.

When you share your story, you challenge the thoughts inside that bid you to hide and isolate yourself. You're directly disobeying your addiction and building up your courage muscle. When you're accepted, loved and embraced with kindness in response, it's even better.

Your inner addict draws from your past experiences and (false) core beliefs to say 'If anyone found out about your struggle, they would judge, reject and be disgusted by you'. That's why we keep it such a secret, isn't it? When you share your story, and receive acceptance and love, it directly challenges that manipulative line that addiction feeds you. You get a chance to see those thoughts aren't always in line with reality. As a sigh of relief floods through you, your fundamental beliefs about yourself, the world and your relationships alter. When you receive grace from a fellow person, it also becomes easier to comprehend the magnificent divine grace that God offers each of us. Sharing your story has profound impacts on your physical, emotional and spiritual experience. This is the reversal of the addiction tree. By revealing your vulnerabilities, and shedding light on your distorted beliefs, you uproot all that is toxic and create an environment where new life can flourish.

Sharing your story is not only an antidote to shame when done carefully, and received by a safe person, but has the power to uplift and liberate others. The secret that has you in shackles may well be the same as your neighbour, the woman sitting behind you in church, the stranger online or even a close friend or family member. My best friend struggled with pornography, too. But both of us kept our lips zipped on it! Until we were honest with each other, we missed out on years of moral support and healing.

We may not all be public speakers, bold storytellers or even confident in the slightest—but you hold a powerful testimony in your heart, sister. And I know when the time is right, God will prompt you, and give you the courage to speak.

Sharing your story may be the last thing you feel like doing. I know, that's the whole reason you're reading this chapter. You're drowning in feelings of shame. Revealing the thing you're most ashamed about to someone doesn't sound very intuitive. But it's all about challenging that shame. So how do you do it?

Sometimes, it will be organic. You won't need a set of instructions—when it just feels right and God has ordained a conversation, you'll just speak from the heart. Other times, it may take some intentionality and planning.

The following is an exercise to help you write out your story to be shared. This can help you get a grip on your own journey (it can be long and complicated!) and filter out the stuff that doesn't need to be shared, or could be unhelpful. I know you could talk about your story all day—I could too. It can be incredibly helpful to write out your entire, detailed story for your own healing, but when it comes to inviting another person (or persons) in, it's best to keep it to a manageable length.

Marnie Ferree in *A L.I.F.E Guide (Women)* outlines how to share your story in principle seven, exercise one[4] (p158-159). She borrows from Alcoholics Anonymous' tradition which encourages people when sharing their story to focus on three things: 'Experience, Strength and Hope'. Their working outline is 'What it was like; what happened; and what it's like now'. These simple guides are helpful for organising your testimony. Ferree uses the following suggestions to flesh out your story:

What it was like

a) **Your sexual history**. You may include any elements of trauma that you experienced, but keep this portion brief and do not give graphic detail. Avoid blaming others or detailing anything triggering for fellow addicts. Do your best to take responsibility for your actions. Include a generalised overview of your acting out history (e.g. masturbating, watching porn) and outline how much time or money you spent on these behaviours.
b) **Your efforts to stop**. Describe various attempts to stop and share why they didn't work out. Include your emotional reaction to these events. Be honest about any level of spiritual or emotional immaturity or errors that played a part in your failure to get sober.
c) **Your consequences**. Outline the major consequences you experienced due to your addiction.

What happened

a) **Your rock bottom**. What finally got your attention enough to seek help?
b) **Your surrender**. Detail the day you really made the decision to get well and surrender your life of addiction. Share the emotions that accompanied this.

c) **Your journey**. What has your healing journey been like? What are some of the significant moments and emotions?

What it's like now

a) **Your current life**. Describe how your life is different today than when you were acting out or when your struggle was at its peak. What's changed? What improvements do you see? What have you learned about yourself, God and community?
b) **Your gratitude**. Share what you're grateful for: spiritually, emotionally, physically, specific people or events. Mention the gifts you've found in recovery.

Where do I share? Who do I tell?

Make a list of people you might like to share your story with. Start small, and when you feel confident you can increase your audience if you wish. Don't rush yourself and avoid running around town spilling your story upon everyone. That would probably be pushing some healthy boundaries. Your story is sacred and should be shared with people who are safe. You don't have to limit sharing your journey with only women who may have sexual struggles, either. The amazing thing about sharing your story is that it can be transformational for so many people. You'll probably find that even people who haven't struggled with sex addiction can relate to your experience of shame, powerlessness and trauma. Those going through mental health issues, divorce, other substance addictions and grief may well relate to your journey and see hope through your choice to recover, get support and be vulnerable in sharing.

Sharing your personal journey of recovery or ongoing struggle with pornography is also an amazing tool for changing culture. You heard me right, your story can change the world! We all know that porn is wrongly considered a guy's issue. Most of us have probably sifted through male recovery resources hoping for a feminine voice, or sat through a sermon on lust and left frustrated that it was directed at men. Both the Church and the secular world have ignored women who struggle with sex for too long. Part of the problem is the silence. Your story has the power to smash through stigma and silence. Your boldness can bring awareness for other women. It can educate male leaders and the culture of your church. Bringing female porn addiction into the light is a glorious and worthy cause to share your story. Join me in fighting the culture of shame and secrecy by bravely proclaiming your struggle and story! It's time for a revolution.

Below are some suggestions of where to start sharing:

- Your accountability partner is a great start.
- Are you in a twelve-step or recovery support group (online or in real life)? Ask if you can share your story there.
- Your counsellor.
- A close friend.
- If you feel brave, you can post a video or blog online.
- You may want to share with a wider audience like a church group or Bible study. Testimonies are always appreciated.
- The Grace Spot has a 'share your story' section for this very purpose, it can even be anonymous.

Service

Alcoholics Anonymous list 'service' as their twelfth and final step for participants. This service is based on the knowledge gained from the previous eleven steps, and their personal experiences throughout recovery. At a twelve-step meeting, it is very common to find more experienced members mentoring and serving those who are new. They devote time to accountability, checking-in, listening to shared inventories and being available for counselling in times of crisis or crossroads.

Service is part of recovery.

Service isn't a thirteenth step for when you've got it all together completely. It's not something you just come back to do once addiction is no longer part of your life—it actually helps you heal. Service crushes shame.

This book is primarily about pornography addiction, not alcoholism. But the tenets of AA are remarkably similar to sexual recovery—they're all addictions, right? This is particularly true when it comes to the twelfth step.

Service towards other struggling women is a win-win situation. They get the support they need, and you reap the benefits as well. A relevant aphorism says 'if you help someone up the hill, you get closer yourself'. This is so true of the recovery journey. When you serve others in their healing, you gain a deep sense of purpose and fulfilment. As you minister to other women dealing with inner shame, you also gain perspective and insight.

You realise you really aren't the only one who feels unworthy or lost. You learn that porn is the enemy, not yourself. You come to see you are not the worst person in the world; neither is your sister in recovery. Through service, you will realise we all make different mistakes in life, but they don't define us. By walking alongside your struggling sisters, you will gain inspiration, motivation and strength to continue your own healing journey. Serving other female addicts also teaches you about self-compassion. When a friend or fellow recovery warrior confides their personal shame to you, or confesses a lapse, your gut reaction will be to love them. Recovering women have a great capacity for love. Your heart will be moved to comfort, console and challenge their self-loathing words; you will encourage them and reassure them of their worth. This is great practice for when it comes to self-talk, and having perspective on your own struggles. When you feel shame impending, stop for a moment and ask yourself 'would I say this to a friend in the same situation?'. By speaking shameless truth over others struggling in a similar way to you, you'll begin to see the inconsistencies in your own thinking towards yourself, and hopefully be able to take the words you've been speaking over others, and apply them to yourself.

Helping one another heal is such a vulnerable act, and this is the crucible where true intimacy and friendship are forged. These things are the antidote to shame.

Service doesn't have to be limited to walking with other recovering women, though. You may not have many other struggling women in your circle (or perhaps you do, but just don't know it).

Acts of service can be big, small or mediocre; they can be done anywhere. Perhaps an elderly woman needs help carrying her groceries or figuring out the self-serve check-out, maybe you return a lost dog to its owner or give a few dollars to a local homeless man. You could do grander things, such as volunteering at a local shelter, animal rescue, church or soup kitchen. If you have a specific area of interest, engage with that by serving; it could be supporting a charity which works with poverty-stricken children, environmental groups or fostering abandoned animals. It can be anything that draws your heart. All these things give a sense of purpose and positivity. They're also great ways to re-engage with the world and to restore intimacy with community.

Not only this but serving makes you feel good. Giving back is satisfying and empowering. It's a great way to get outside of your own head for a while and explore your capabilities. It might even become a regular hobby! Serving makes you feel good, and the better you feel, the less you want to escape reality.

A gentle warning

Service in recovery is not, and should not become, a form of self-flagellation. You're not serving to make up for your sins, justify bad behaviours or hide your short-comings. Overdoing it on ministry commitments or donating a few extra dollars into the charity box aren't going to earn you good karma points, or genuinely remove your shame. Trust me, punishing yourself only makes room for more shame and exhaustion—both of which fuel the addiction cycle.

You don't need punishment; Jesus took the final punishment on the cross. His sacrifice was enough to earn you a place in heaven, to take away your sins. Period. He said 'It is finished'. Service then, is about joy and healing, not crucifying yourself over and over for your sexual (or other) sins. Ask God where he'd have you serve, where your gifts can be utilised and you can heal alongside others. And don't forget to instil boundaries. You can be a good, and worthy and motivated woman without saying yes to everything. Know your limits and abilities. Churches and charities often get overexcited with offers of service and overburden volunteers and dry out their love and service stores.

Service done out of obligation, fear or punishment isn't healing for anyone.

Conclusion

As you finish this chapter, I want you to feel empowered to stand up against shame. Even in the smallest of ways, know you are capable. You are capable of sharing your story, of serving others and of using your voice to break stigma and make a change in culture and in your own heart. You can be transformed from someone silenced by shame into someone who bravely speaks out. From someone whose hands have been wrung raw by the rope that binds you to shame into someone who joyfully cares for herself and others. I want you to look shame in the face and say 'I'm fighting back!'. Practice these activities and build that courage muscle, and soon your brain will rewire itself so the simplest route will be from mistake to self-love. Shame can be overcome.

Action Steps:

1. **Use the outline under the heading 'Overcoming shame is also about sharing your story' to prepare a ten to fifteen-minute talk, or 1000-2000-word article, about your story of addiction and recovery. You might also want to write a longer story for your own records; it can help to understand yourself and gain clarity on the messy journey.**
2. **Consider who you might be able to share your story with and pursue this when you're ready.**

3. **Brainstorm and write down ways you can serve others, either in recovery or in general. It doesn't have to be big—maybe you can set a goal to do the dishes at home more often or help a struggling friend. You might want to contact a local charity or church to offer your services, too.**

FINAL WORDS

You made it to the end of the book! Hooray! Good on you. How do you feel? You may be feeling a little overwhelmed. I've just spent the last sixty thousand words dropping loads of information on you, some of which may be totally new and may go against what you've previously been taught about women, sex, porn and recovery. It's a lot. I know you might also be feeling a little scared. Maybe you even feel worse than when you picked up this book because you've seen all the work it takes to find freedom. This process takes all the time it needs, and involves unravelling and undoing everything you've been living. Yikes.

I'm praying there's also a sense of hope stirring within you, too. I hope everything you've read has pushed back on the lies you've been told: that porn is a 'guys issue', that you're alone, that you're unworthy of love and freedom. I hope you've found some bravery within yourself after reading the stories of other women and how it is possible to overcome pornography, and that you feel there is a future for you. One full of love, joy and relationship. A future where the screen no longer commands your heart but has made way for courage.

Whatever condition your heart is in at this point, you need to make a choice. After all this reading and reflecting, some action is needed if you haven't already jumped into the process. This is your fork in the road.

You know you have a problem with porn, you now know the process needed to overcome it and restore yourself. You've been provided with action steps and the practical tools needed to begin this amazing journey. What are you going to do with this? You can run and hide, ignoring the problem like you've been doing for a while now. You can continue trying to push through in your recovery without dealing with the underlying issues and remain shackled to secrecy and shame. You can avoid the scary stuff like vulnerability, honesty and reconnecting with people and continue to live your life as it currently is.

Or, you can fully give yourself to recovery. To be afraid but brave and commit to doing the hard work outlined in this book. You can choose to invest in your healing and create a better future for yourself and those around you, with support and the resources you need to keep yourself afloat. You can make the safe choice, or the brave one. It's up to you.

I hope you dig deep and find your courage. The decision to invest in recovery will change your life. It might even make long-lasting generational change in your family. The best gift you can give your future babies is the gift of a healed mamma. Pain travels through families until someone is willing to feel it. Choose to feel it so your children and their children don't need to.

As you bravely set out upon this journey to healing and restoration, remember this is a process and you will make mistakes. That's okay! There are definite steps you must take in order to put yourself in a place of recovery, but it won't be as simple as following step one through to ten and winning the recovery game. You will experience set-backs, of both your own and others' creation, you'll come up against hairy topics that make you run away and hide for a little while, life circumstances can change and the unpredictability of life can turn your recovery upside down at a moment's notice. You might need to re-start your recovery many times over, or re-visit certain practices such as accountability or inventory. This book was written to be read over and over—consider it like a preventative asthma puffer, rather than a single dose miracle cure. Keep coming back to it, and go deeper every time. Over the years, I bailed out on accountability and tracking my recovery a number of times. I simply faded away and quietly relapsed. Maybe it wasn't always so quiet ... a few times upsetting life circumstances just made me mad and I said 'Screw it! I don't care about freedom anymore!'

These were the times when I had to come back to that choice point all over again. Do I want to hide it out and stay safe, or put the hard yards in to overcome? It's not these set-backs that define you or your recovery but the courage to get back up, be honest and start again.

Recovery is a marathon. Actually, an ultra-marathon might be more accurate. I want you to impress this fact on your heart as you start the race. Give this your all, but if (or rather when) set-backs or lapses occur, remember you don't have to go back to the starting line all over again. Just like if you were to stumble over a rock during a race, simply pick yourself up, brush off the dirt and keep running. You're not at war or in a video game. A slip-up doesn't equal a 'game over'—it's just part of reality, another opportunity to learn from your mistake and grow.

I'm still on the journey with you, sister. People may look at me and see the picture of recovery. I've written a book, I speak at events and share my story without hesitation. Generally, I'm free from compulsive pornography use and the shame that accompanies it. I'm recovered. This doesn't mean I'm perfect or have always chosen wisely when it comes to temptation. Sure, I'm no longer compulsively drawn to sexual content and live a happy and fulfilled life full of relationships, but I've messed up too. Even while running The Grace Spot and blogging about recovery, I've faltered. As I wrote this book, I was drawn into watching porn and letting sexual fantasies creep in. I can't say I've been totally porn-free for five years. I wish I could, it all sounds so heroic and inspiring. Wouldn't that be the best way to end a book on porn addiction recovery? I suppose it might be inspiring, but it's not reality and maybe that's what you need more than a picture of perfection to strive for. Failure is part of the journey. I've learned, grown and I continue to do so. Perfection isn't the end-goal of recovery, but grace and wisdom are.

You'll give yourself the best chance of full recovery if you head right back to chapter two and dig into every chapter, doing the Action Steps and activities outlined. However, if you do nothing else from this book, I want you to remember these five tenets.

1. Restrict

Get yourself motivated for the journey by doing a purge. Get rid of any porn or triggering material you have access to. This means deleting anything you may have saved, throwing out magazines or books, deleting online accounts where you act out, downloading filtering software and even taking a break from social media if you need. When it comes to your socials, at least go through all your accounts and delete or block any person or account that shares sexual content. An alternative option is to ditch the smart phone entirely and buy a cheap 'dumb-phone' without internet access.

Annoying, but works a treat. Doing a full porn-purge is empowering. It almost feels like setting all the ex-boyfriend's things on fire in a break-up rage. Exciting and healing.

2. Get support

You need people! If you choose to try and do this on your own, you're really choosing not to recover. You need an accountability partner or group to pull you out of the depths of temptation when it hits, you need a cheer squad to celebrate your victories with and to act as sounding boards for your future plans. Not only do you need official accountability support, but simply having close friends to distract your mind and have fun with is so important to recovery. Remember, this isn't all about restriction, but restoration too. A professional therapist or mentor is also a very wise investment as you seek to uncover the 'why' behind your struggle and deal with the strong emotions that come up in recovery.

3. Track

Track your progress! Get motivated by finding yourself a nice tracking system, either as an app or a physical paper calendar. Remember, counting 'days since' isn't helpful—use a tracking option that allows you to record both slip-ups and victories. Head to The Grace Spot and download the worksheets from chapters three, five and six. Print them off or fill them in digitally to help you get a better understanding of your personal struggle and needs. Having these in a visible place can help you remain motivated to pursue freedom in times of temptation.

4. Journal and create

Express yourself. Whatever your medium may be—journaling, poetry, music, art or anything else—find a way to creatively express your feelings. Doing so provides space for reflection, processing and planning. These are all vital aspects when it comes to healing emotional pain. Perhaps you can mark the beginning of this journey by buying yourself a nice new journal or artbook.

5. Seek restoration. Don't focus on avoiding porn.

Choose one hobby, project or friendship to invest in while you do the hard work of recovery. It's important to have interests and goals in life that have nothing to do with your recovery. Spending every moment of your day thinking about porn (whether it's about using porn or not using porn) can be triggering in itself, if not totally depressing. Pick something you can focus on that will bring you joy and restoration.

No matter how messed up your past or present seems, the woman struggling with pornography and shame can live happily ever after. You can find healing; you can overcome pornography and the obsessive behaviours that hinder your potential. You can learn how to be vulnerable and relearn trust, you can experience true intimacy in relationship with others, God and yourself. You can rebuild what has been broken and create a new life for yourself and those you love. You can be restored.

CONTACT

You are welcome to contact Alice for further support, advice, to ask questions or simply share your story with a woman who gets it. She is also available to speak at your conference, event, school or church on a range of topics relating to women and pornography, including training leaders to be equipped with the tools and knowledge to minister to the women in their care.

Website: thegracespot.com
Email: alice@thegracespot.com
Facebook: facebook.com/thegracespotministries
Twitter: twitter.com/GSpotMinistries
Instagram: instagram.com/thegspot_ministries

RESOURCES MENTIONED

Because resources update regularly, please visit The Grace Spot website for up-to-date information.

ACKNOWLEDGEMENTS

Mum. Thank you for reading to me from such a young age and instilling a love of words within me. You taught me the importance of sharing stories, and I'm thankful for your continual encouragement of my writing, from the earliest age—even though it was sometimes on the wall ... written in lipstick—and throughout the writing of *Restored*.

Lukas. Thank you for everything. For the years of friendship and fun before we were a couple, the wise advice and kindness, for making me break up with the boy from chapter one, for protecting me, always being generous without any expectation of something in return, for your endless patience and understanding of things that were foreign to you: my trauma, fears, history and family wounds. God placed you in my life to be an agent of change and healing. Before we knew our lives would be eternally entwined, He was working through you and making you part of my story; part of my healing. This book wouldn't exist without you, because my healing wouldn't be complete without you.

Thank you for always being there to listen to me and wipe away my tears. Thank you for listening to me talk about the book, for letting me read it out loud for hours and sharing your input. My favourite quote from *Restored* is actually one of your lines. I should give you commission. You've always believed whole-heartedly in the vision and mission of this ministry. Your encouragement has been an endless source of courage and motivation through the tough times. Thank you for not being afraid of dating and marrying a vocal ex-porn addict with a backlog of emotional issues. You are an answered prayer and an enormous blessing. (P.S. Thanks for working so I can stay at home and write about porn all day, every day. You're the best!)

Mel. You're the first person I ever told about my struggle, and the best friend I've ever had. Without you, I wouldn't have recovered. No matter the distance between us, you will always be my number one, my sister and another answered prayer from our amazing God. You kept me honest and accountable for so many years and with the perfect amount of gentleness and butt-kicking, you helped me heal. You asked me the hard questions. You were honest and real with me. You offered me so much love and kindness and celebrated my victories with me in the best ways! Do you remember when we went on that hiking picnic to celebrate one hundred days of freedom from porn? I'll never forget the fun we had exploring and breaking that vine swing! You are my safe place, my cheerleader and inspiration. Thank you for always being willing to share your own story and be part of The Grace Spot. You're the kind of woman anyone would be blessed to have on their team. And I'm so glad you're on mine!

Katie & Elise. You have both stood by my side and kept me accountable in times of temptation, and offered unconditional love and comfort in times of trouble. You are both precious gifts from God, and I am thankful for your friendship and willingness to share in the vulnerabilities of life with me. You have both been huge supporters of The Grace Spot and *Restored*. Thank you for believing in me, and reminding me of the goodness and sovereignty of Jesus when anxiety tries to punch me in the face.

Marnie Ferree, Jessica Harris & Crystal Renaud. Thank you for going ahead of me and laying out a path for healing specifically for women. Without your courage and wisdom, my healing would have been so much more painful and confusing, and taken so much longer. Thank you for fighting for and creating recovery resources that used feminine pronouns, for giving me hope that I wasn't the only woman struggling with porn and that I could recover. You not only provided me with the support I needed to break free, but inspired me to share my own story and write *Restored* despite all the challenges I faced.

Anglicare Counselling. I will never forget the healing that occurred in those tidy little rooms in Wollongong all those years ago. For over ten years I attended counselling at Anglicare and it changed my life. As I dealt with trauma, anxiety, depression, relationship breakdowns, guilt, family woundedness, pornography addiction, shame, chronic illness and planning for the future, Anna and Eileen were there for me. They genuinely cared and gave every effort to loving me and providing me with the best professional therapy. I felt the love of God in both of those women, and it changed me. My work with Anglicare has been integral to my healing and being able to look back and gather the lessons learned for *Restored*. These two women and the ministry of Anglicare will forever be a huge part of my story, and I owe them all my gratitude for helping me get to where I am today.

Lacy. This book wouldn't exist without your tenacity, encouragement and the hours you spent talking me through the process of writing, publishing and listening to my confused rants and questions. It was such a blessing to have a wiser, older woman who had gone before me in recovery and publishing by my side, cheering me on. Seriously, I tried for so long to get this book done and it wasn't until you said 'sit down, write and don't edit!' that it became reality. Thank you for helping me fulfil my dream of becoming an author.

Johanna. You are a miracle worker. I am deeply grateful for your editing services. Thank you for dedicating so much time to reading through every word of *Restored*, for being another set of eyes and making my words so much clearer. Your editing was artful, and so needed. You were so kind to me in your encouragement, in correcting my spelling and structural errors and polishing *Restored* so it truly came to life. This book is insurmountably better because of you.

Saffron and Co. Creative. Thank you for creating a beautiful cover for *Restore*d. From the very first meeting we had, I felt like the team understood and celebrated my vision, jumping on board with enthusiasm. Saffron and Carmela, I owe it to your stunning cover design for grabbing many women's attention so they would actually pick up this book and get to the healing words inside. Thank you for bringing my book baby to life in a spectacular way.

The Facebook Prayer Support Group and TGS Ultra Support Group. To the eighty-odd people who joined my prayer groups all those years ago, who have continued to read my constant status updates and pray faithfully for this ministry, thank you! I am so grateful for this faithful group who wanted to know what was happening, who were invested in this ministry and who gave their time to encourage me and pray for everything I posted (which was a lot, sorry guys). It means the world to have this support.

Financial Donors. So many amazing people have given generously to support The Grace Spot and *Restored*. I have been blown away by the way people have provided for me over the years. From large one-off donations, to regular monthly gifts, I have been so incredibly blessed. A number of friends, family and even strangers contributed to my fundraiser to attend the Coalition to End Sexual Exploitation Global Summit in the U.S in 2018. The connections I made there were integral to me being able to publish *Restored,* so for those who supported me on that journey, I thank you too! You are part of this book's story. Thank you for giving generously and being part of the creation of *Restored*. Thank you for partnering with me to develop this resource and reduce the shame and stigma that women struggling with pornography face every day.

The women who share their stories. Many women have shared their stories with me, and given me permission to share them in this book and on The Grace Spot. They are brave and inspiring people. To every woman who has had the guts to share her story, thank you. You minister to me on my darkest days and remind me I am not alone.

You inspire me, and have made this book so much stronger and more powerful. I hope sharing your story has made you feel stronger, too.

Jesus. You did this. You stood by me, healed me and loved me. You gave me the opportunity to write this book and share it with the world. People might hear my story and think'where was God when her life turned to shit?' I wondered that too for a while, when everything hurt. But looking back, I wouldn't change a thing. Struggling with addiction (and all the other painful things that led me there) sucked, but through it you gave me my dream: to become an author, to speak, write and break stigma for women. You used my pain to make me into the woman I always prayed I would be. I don't care about the pain anymore, because what others intended for evil, you used for good!

REFERENCES

CHAPTER TWO: ACCOUNTABILITY

[1] Riordan A. Longing for Intimacy [Internet] [cited 2019 Sept 4]. Available from: Longingforintimacy.com

[2] Fortify [Internet]. Fortify, 2017. [Cited 2019 Oct 14]. Available from https://www.joinfortify.com/

CHAPTER THREE: INVENTORY

[1] Crabbe MJ. Body Positive Power. London: Vermilion; 2017.

[2] Bacon L. Health at Every Size: the surprising truth about your weight. US: BenBella Books; 2010.

CHAPTER FOUR: THE MASTURBATION CONTROVERSY

[1] Carnes P. Out of The Shadows: understanding sexual addiction. 3rd ed. Center City, Minnesota: Hazelden; 2001. 189 P.

CHAPTER FIVE: UNDERSTANDING YOUR ADDICTION CYCLE

[1] Ferree MC. No Stones: women redeemed from sexual addiction. 2nd ed. Downers Grove: InterVarsity Press; 2010. 47-50 p.

[2] Bethesda Workshops [Internet]. Nashville, TN, Bethesda Workshops, 2019. [cited 2019 Oct 2]. Available from: https://www.bethesdaworkshops.org/

[3] World Health Organisation. ICD-11 for mortality and morbidity statistics [Internet]. WHO, 2019 [cited 2019 Oct 3]. Available from: https://icd.who.int/browse11/l m/en#/http%3a%2f%2fid.who.int%2ficd%2fentity%2f1630268048

[4] Fight The New Drug. How porn affects the brain [Internet]. Fight The New Drug Inc. 2019 [cited 2019 Oct 14]. Available from: https://fightthenewdrug.org/how-porn-can-become-addictive/

[5] Doidge N. The Brain that Changes Itself: stories of personal triumph from the frontiers of brain science. Carlton North, Vic: Scribe Publications; 2010.

[6] Carnes P. Out of The Shadows: understanding sexual addiction. 3rd ed. Center City, Minnesota: Hazelden; 2001.

[7]Ferree MC. No Stones: women redeemed from sexual addiction. 2nd ed. Downers Grove: InterVarsity Press; 2010

CHAPTER SIX: REFLECTION

[1] Brownlee P. Dance With Me in the Heart: the adults' guide to great infant-parent partnerships. Revised ed. Thames, New Zealand: Good Egg Books; 2016.

[2] Carnes P. Out of The Shadows: understanding sexual addiction. 3rd ed. Center City, Minnesota: Hazelden; 2001.

[3] Ferree MC. No Stones: women redeemed from sexual addiction. 2nd ed. Downers Grove: InterVarsity Press; 2010.

[4] Brand R. Recovery: freedom from our addictions. London: Bluebird; 2017.

[5] White Ribbon Australia. Types of abuse [Internet]. [cited 2019 Nov 2]. Available from https://www. whiteribbon.org.au/understand-domestic-violence/types-of-abuse/

CHAPTER SEVEN: WHAT NOW? HEALING YOUR PAIN AND TRAUMA

[1] Ferree MC. No Stones: women redeemed from sexual addiction. 2nd ed. Downers Grove: InterVarsity Press; 2010.193 p.

CHAPTER TEN: OVERCOMING SHAME

[1] Brown B. Shame V. Guilt [Internet]. 2019. [cited 2019 Oct 2]. Available from: https://brenebrown.com/blog/2013/01/14/shame-v-guilt/

[2] Brown B. Daring Greatly: How the courage to be vulnerable transforms the way we live, love, parent and lead. New York: Gotham Books; 2012. 53 p.

[3] Scheff T. The Ubiquity of Hidden Shame in Modernity. *Cultural Sociology* [Internet]. 2014 Feb [Cited 2019 Nov 2]; *8*(2), 129–141.Available from: https://doi.org/10.1177/1749975513507244

[4] Ferree MC. A L.I.F.E Guide. USA: Freedom Everyday LLC; 2007. 158-159 p.

Milton Keynes UK
Ingram Content Group UK Ltd.
UKHW021319160124
436126UK00029B/1623

9 780648 72